Selling to the Pain

Closing More Deals in Healthcare Sales

Dr. Tom R. McDougal, Jr.
CEO and Founder
Gylen Castle, LLC

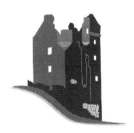

Selling to the Pain

Copyright © 2016 by Gylen Castle, LLC

Gylen Castle, LLC
22 Inverness Center Parkway, Suite 160
Birmingham, Alabama 35242
info@gylencastle.com

Printed in the United States of America

First Edition

Acknowledgements

I have humbly realized that writing a book is a major challenge. While I have trained nearly a thousand individuals related to our strategies for effective healthcare sales strategy, converting that training to a book is a very different task.

I am very grateful to my mentors, hospital leadership teams, colleagues, and the many clients of Gylen Castle that have shaped my thoughts on what works and what does not work in sales strategy. I also appreciate the many subject matter experts that have produced hundreds of books on leadership, sales, and efficiency. You have also shaped my opinions, whether I agreed with you or not.

My family has been very supportive during this writing process. To my children, Mary Ann and Madden, don't ever let someone tell you that you cannot accomplish a dream. Dream big, work harder, stay focused. I am thankful to Emily Thompson for your assistance in reviewing, formatting and and proofing this book. To Mary Chaput, thank you for your inspiration for the book title – it is perfect.

To those of you that want to increase your sales effectiveness and efficiency and achieve higher Close Rates, this book is for you.

Selling to the Pain

Table of Contents

Selling to the Pain

Closing More Deals in Healthcare Sales

Dr. Tom R. McDougal, Jr.
CEO and Founder
Gylen Castle, LLC

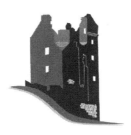

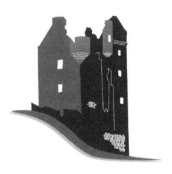

Introduction: Why Did I Say "No"?

In 2003, I was serving as the CEO of a hospital that was part of a large and successful system of hospitals located across the country. Our hospital Vice President had met with a sales professional from a company that wanted to sell a service to our hospital. The "pitch" the Vice President had heard peaked his interest and he had presented the concept to me in a quick five-minute discussion. I was curious about the opportunity so I agreed to listen to a presentation from the sales professional.

The presentation was well done as the sales professional had prepared, completed his research, and was succinct in the presentation. The pitch was a technology opportunity for our hospital projected to add an estimated $500,000 in new revenue and $100,000 in profit to our bottom line. The margin for the new service was acceptable given current hospital margins. Additionally, the sales professional believed the hospital would gain $70,000 in profitability from improved efficiency of operations. However, these numbers were soft and it would be difficult to verify if the projected performance resulted from this solution.

After hearing this presentation of a seemingly good opportunity, I told the sales professional that we were not interested in pursuing the opportunity. The look of surprise was clear on the faces of the Vice President and the sales professional. And, with that "no" the meeting ended as did the opportunity for the sales professional to sell his solution to the hospital.

The next day when meeting with the Vice President, he asked about my decision the prior day to decline to pursue the opportunity. I admit that I did not have a good answer. On the surface, the opportunity looked logical but my gut was telling me differently. I was bothered that I could not explain my reasoning to the Vice President. The problem I had was that I really did not understand why I declined to pursue the opportunity.

For the coming ten years I would study, research, and try to understand the decision process in hospital c-suites and large organizations. I saw companies and sales professionals struggling with their Close Rates and gaining access to decision makers.

My realization was the sales strategy most companies use when selling to healthcare organizations is simply not working as it did in the past. Traditional methods for sales have changed little over the past 25 years yet the culture of business decision making in healthcare organizations has changed dramatically. The types of leaders in the c-suite are different and tenure for decision makers is shorter than it has been in history. Thus, a culture of "team decisions" has emerged. Companies must now focus on the customer and a strategy of *Selling to the Pain.*

In 2013, I formed Gylen Castle as a sales strategy boutique advisory firm to tackle the problem that really boiled down to sales inefficiency. Our narrow niche is to work with companies that sell products or services to hospitals and healthcare providers. We have worked with all types of companies over the years. Clients include a wide variety from software-as-a-service technology firms to construction firms, but they all have the same goal to improve their Close Rates to grow revenue more efficiently.

The sizes of our clients have ranged from startup companies that have zero in sales to date to companies that have sold billions the previous year such as STERIS and the GE Capital Healthcare Division. As a result of this wide range of company sizes, we have worked with CEOs that handle all of the sales to companies that have well established and large complex sales teams. Gylen Castle is very unique due to our narrow niche and the variety of companies that fall in that niche.

At the core of Gylen Castle is our fundamental strategy for sales efficiency by focusing on the client need. I have researched the market and understand both the hospital decision-maker side and the challenges companies face when selling to hospitals. The *Selling to the Pain* strategy is proven and works for all companies based on our four principle components:

1. Effectively navigating a complicated decision process;

2. Utilizing Value Proposition Messaging to identify the pain an organization is experiencing in terms of performance and communicate strategies that drive improvement results;

3. The Decision Table to understand the factors affecting decisions and how and when a decision is made; and

4. Accountability Sales to hold the decision maker accountable to listen, act, and help you close the deal.

During the past three years, our work has included many training programs for company leaders and sales professionals. Increasingly, I have been asked if there was a book that reinforced our training materials and could be a leave behind resource for maintaining focus. This book is a result of that request and is designed to serve as both a pre-training primer and a post-training supplement to our client-focused advisement. This book can also stand on its own without training.

The information contained within this book is valuable to your company. It is a roadmap to the principle strategies and components that will improve your performance. As with any strategy, success is found in devising a plan that is executable if you want your company to truly change and grow. I strongly advise that you use these principles once they are shaped around your company culture, what you are selling, and to whom you are selling. This book of our training principles is a great primer to understand and navigate a difficult sales environment.

There are four sections to this book. First, I address why selling in the current decision culture has become so difficult. Second, I discuss the decision process and the application of The Decision Table to unpack the factors affecting decisions. Third, Accountability Sales will explain the strategy for increasing your Close Rate whereby you learn to hold the decision maker accountable to help you close the deal. Fourth and finally, I address some of the sales strategy fundamentals that I did not want to include in the first three sections to keep the readability time to a minimum. If we are working to improve the efficiency of sales, or anything else for that matter, the book certainly should not be long.

As a final note, this book is written and based on strategies and experiences from sales in healthcare. However, our principles and strategies transfer over to selling in other industries that have large complex organizations. These industries include banking, insurance, technology, service, education, non-profit, and even government organizations. Each of these industries share a number of commonalities with healthcare including:

- Administrative functions in the c-suite overseeing a large workforce;

- Complex authority and decision making structures;

- Powerful individuals within the organization that have a strong voice but limited decision authority; and

- Long sales cycles to make purchase decisions.

The leaders of Gylen Castle are experts in sales strategies to improve Close Rates. That is the metric that matters. Our techniques are proven and can provide valuable insight to a broader range of industries. If you are frustrated with sales challenges, the principles of this book can help you improve your sales effectiveness and efficiency. Let's get started.

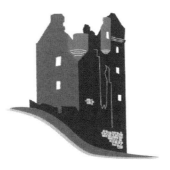

Section 1: Why is Healthcare Sales so Freakin' Difficult?

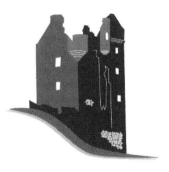

Chapter 1: Look Here, Big Boy

This chapter is not a biography. However, to understand my recommendations and strategies related to sales, you need to understand the background and experiences that shaped my conclusions. And, you will probably get a good laugh in the process related to events I have experienced.

I received my Bachelor of Science degree in 1991 from the Brock School of Business at Samford University and then enrolled at UAB for the dual degree track of a Master of Science in Healthcare Administration (MSHA) degree and a Master of Business

Administration (MBA) degree. The reason for two Master degrees was simple – Rush Jordan. I had been accepted to the MSHA program at UAB. Mr. Jordan was a member of the Healthcare Hall of Fame and a leader in the MSHA program. My father was a veteran healthcare leader and Mr. Jordan had been his boss years before. So, I had the family connection and I knew Mr. Jordan well. At the MSHA orientation, Mr. Jordan said, "Mr. McDougal, you will be enrolling in the dual degree program, correct?" I responded as everyone responded to Mr. Jordan, "Yes, sir." I then left his office to find out what the heck a "dual degree program" was and to sign up.

Two years later, I had completed the classroom portion of the MSHA/MBA dual degree program. Part of the MSHA program was a required full time residency for 9-12 months following the course work. I interviewed with a lot of great hospitals and healthcare systems and landed at Baptist Health System of South Carolina, now part of Palmetto Health Alliance.

Chuck Beaman, CEO for Baptist, was my mentor and took me under his wing. I had chosen well as Chuck was really good to me. He is a jovial and highly intelligent person that understands the art of leadership. I was smart enough to listen to him.

I spent the first year in an official residency position and then Chuck offered for me to join the team long term as Director of Business Development and Planning. I had the opportunity to be involved in many important initiatives including our affiliate provider network development including hospitals and physician practices. In this role, I was involved in affiliations and acquisitions and really developed an understanding of how hospitals and healthcare organizations function as businesses. I have been known to say that hospitals are businesses on steroids. The complexity of reimbursement for services provided and the necessity of physician referrals for business volume make healthcare more challenging than any other industry.

One of my primary roles was to develop affiliation relationships between Baptist and surrounding small town community hospitals. Following the second hospital affiliation deal, I presented the contract to Chuck, he signed it quickly and slid the agreement across the table to me. With a big smile, he asked, "What day do you want to start?" I honestly had no idea what he was talking about.

A few weeks later I was CEO of Barnwell County Hospital in rural South Carolina at age 27. To say I was green would be generous. The truth is I had no idea what I was doing. I had never run an operating department of a hospital as I had been on the corporate side. I was fortunate that Chuck shared with me what he liked to call "Pearls of Wisdom." For three years, it had not been unusual for Chuck to call me into his office with "McDougal, come in here. I want to drop a 'pearl' on you" And, then he would laugh and share valuable insight, most of which I carry with me to this day.

My orientation as a new and young CEO was provided by Chuck. He advised me initially and ongoing related to Board and Physician relations. Orientation also included "Pearls of Widow" such as:

1. "It's ok to say you don't know. But, don't say it frequently"; and
2. "Be seen, but if they see you all the time, they will think you don't have anything to do."

Great advice. Regarding my time in Barnwell, it was an adventure. The hospital was very small at 53 licensed beds. The County owned the hospital and the County Commissioners appointed the Board of Directors for the hospital. Each County Council member could unilaterally appoint one Board member so I had a Board full of individually chosen, politically appointed, and politically motivated members.

The local radio station would attend every open Board meeting and record the meeting by cassette recorder to re-play the discussion on the radio during the next two days. No, that was not comfortable. One month, a Board member called two days after a Board meeting and said, "I don't like what I just heard you say on the radio." He was referring to the recording. I had to remind him that he was in attendance at the meeting and did not have a problem with what I said during the actual Board meeting. Flustered, he blurted out, "But it sounds different on the radio!" Ugh.

The Medical Staff and employees were fantastic. I quickly learned that hospitals present a very challenging environment of the unexpected. As a result, I have experienced many unusual events that are a byproduct of the environment. In other words, crazy things happen.

I managed to survive two years at Barnwell. I use the word "survive" as it was a battle to get the hospital to a profit and to deal with the Board. I really had no idea what I was doing, but fortunately a number of the department managers of the hospital took this "kid" under their wings. Yes, they called me a "kid" and I let them. The clinical department leaders, including Jenny, Trisha, and Fran, invested in me by helping me make good decisions and teaching me about how hospitals really operate. I chose not to hire a Chief Nursing Officer as I wanted all patient care directors and functions to report directly to me as this was the best way to learn operations. That decision has served me well my entire career.

It really is a wonder that I survived. I will always remember a medical staff meeting where we discussed a change by Medicare in how they would pay for laparoscopic cholecystectomies. It was an unexpected topic but I had briefed on the Medicare changes so I participated in the discussion. Unfortunately, I had focused on the business side of this issue, not the medical care side. So, after the meeting I went back to my office and pulled out the medical dictionary so I could recall what surgical procedure was a laparoscopic cholecystectomy. Fran caught me reading and never let me live that down. By the way, a laparoscopic cholecystectomy is a surgical procedure that uses a small incision and scope to remove a diseased gallbladder. No, I will never forget that.

My first Halloween, I agreed to honor the tradition of the hospital staff to dress in Halloween costumes. My mistake. I received a call that our Director of Medical Records was dressed as the Grim Reaper. I had to explain to her that her attire was not appropriate as her office was just outside the surgery department. I did not believe a patient seeing the Grim Reaper after surgery would improve our patient satisfaction scores.

After two years in Barnwell, I was recruited to Community Health System (CHS) as the CEO of LV Stabler Memorial Hospital in Greenville, Alabama. Stabler is really where I learned to be an effective and sustainable CEO leader. While a small town and small hospital, my wife had family in Greenville and I loved my team there. The Medical Staff physicians were relatively easy with whom to work. Following a few tweaks, the management team was talented despite the small setting. Connie, Don, John, Vicki, Eddie, and Joey formed a great team and it was a fun place to work. Most of the time.

Physician recruitment was an adventure in Greenville as a small town environment lacks some of the social activities many physicians desire. The candidates that would consider a small town produces some outstanding physicians and some real characters. For instance, I was threatened by a doctor that he was going to have me killed over a decision to recruit his future competition. I had to fire another doctor twice – once for performance and a second time for having a gun in his hospital campus office during his notice period.

We had a frequent visitor to the hospital who had legally changed his name to "Free Spirit" and he kept us a little on edge. He dressed like Prince after a visit to the local Goodwill store and carried a cane, but had no limp. I had to ask him to leave the hospital one day as he was frightening some of the staff. I wondered during that discussion if that cane would become a weapon. It did not.

Stabler was also the home of the famous story of "Sh-Willie." During a physician's recruitment visit, we met his very interesting fiancé. She bragged on her future husband and stated that he had become a great doctor by nursing their Chihuahua back to health after the dog had been run over by a garbage truck. For that reason, her life long dream was to have a Chihuahua farm.

The dog's name was Sh-Willie. My wife had to ask why. The doctor's fiancé explained that originally the dog's name was Willie but the dog tended to wander around the yard for a longer than normal time before doing his business. So, the doctor would follow him in frustration saying, "Sh*t, Willie! Sh*t, Willie!" They had shortened the name to Sh-Willie. I can't make this stuff up. And, no, we did not recruit the physician.

From Stabler, I was promoted to CEO of Parkway Medical Center in Decatur, Alabama, where I inherited a few superstar leaders and recruited others. The core team was stellar and talented including Steve, Kathy, Sherry, Don, Joel followed by Jim, another Joel, Monty, Brandi, Rahe, Eric, and Bill. Don had followed me to Parkway but the rest of the team was new. Together, they accomplished a great deal. We were fortunate to win a number of CHS National Awards and accomplish some crazy things including a perfect score from a Joint Commission survey. In the light of full disclosure, the team achieved the perfect score. I was just smart enough to recruit and retain the team; and, stay out of their way.

Yes, some crazy things happened at Parkway as well. A visitor committed suicide in the parking lot of the ER. If that was not bad enough, another visitor, rather than our staff, found the poor soul in his car two days later. The media loved that story.

On a bad weather day, the local TV meteorologist announced a funnel cloud was tracking directly to the hospital. I watched the funnel rotate right over the hospital parking lot but it did not touch down in our county.

One bright sunny morning we lost power at the hospital. I suspected a suicide squirrel in a transformer but the cause was a traffic accident. You learn as a hospital executive when the power goes out to count to six as it takes six seconds for the emergency standby generators to start up. The two emergency generators we had in tandem started up as planned. About 15 minutes later, I received a call that generator one had stopped working. I was not too worried as it was a tandem system with double capacity. Five minutes later, the second generator stopped working and in the middle of a weekday morning we had no power. Now, I was worried.

Eric and the maintenance team sprang to action and we had power 22 minutes later, which seemed like an eternity. It took that long as the team had to prime the diesel generators and manually carry fuel from the large outside tank. Amazingly, no patients were harmed and that is an example of just how good that team really was in handling crises and challenges. I am often asked if there were any surgeries in progress during this power outage. We were very fortunate that only one surgery was underway and the surgeon wisely stepped away from the table as he was at a good point to pause the surgery.

For those that are curious, we later learned that a flashlight to check fuel levels in the small tank attached to the generator is not a reliable method. Additionally, when you test run generators you should also test the pump that moves diesel fuel from the main large tank outside to the small tanks on the generators. We had experienced a failure in the pump days or weeks earlier so this particular morning the generators had run out of fuel.

Other crazy things happened during my tenure including losing a psychiatric inpatient as she had disappeared from her room.

That is what I was told – she disappeared like a ghost. We organized a team to search for her and I personally found her on the roof huddled next to an air handling unit. I still don't know how she opened the locked window to climb out onto the roof. We also had an inpatient call 911 one day as she did not think the nurses were responding to the call button fast enough.

One of my favorite doctors at Parkway was a brilliant Internist with his office in a building attached to the hospital. I would visit him regularly and one day he saw me coming and waved me into a patient room. A patient had a bad looking skin wound problem on her lower leg. The physician proceeded to ask me if I thought the medical text book he was holding had a picture matching the woman's skin problem. Without thinking, I looked at several pictures including those on adjacent pages. I then "concurred" that I thought the first picture was correct. The doctor explained the skin condition to the patient and that the treatment would be fairly simple. The patient was so excited that she grabbed me and gave me a hug while saying, "Thank you so much, doctor." Stunned with not knowing how to respond, I said, "You're welcome."

After six great years at Parkway, CHS planned to sell the hospital to another company. I chose to remain with CHS and accepted the CEO position at Springs Memorial Hospital in Lancaster, South Carolina, just outside of Charlotte, North Carolina. The team there was also outstanding including Karen, Julie, Janet, Brit, Elmer, and Cliff. Unfortunately, the economy was terrible as it was the time of the Great Recession. To make matters worse, Lancaster previously was a textile town that now had the last of those jobs moving overseas. If memory serves correct, the county unemployment rate reached 21% during my tenure. I was playing a lot of defense.

The stories at Springs were as amazing as some of the stories at other hospitals during my career. One morning, the Emergency Department Director was upset about her department's performance and suddenly burst into tears in my office. I was shocked. Through the tears she explained, "I am not crying because I am upset, I am crying because I am pissed!" I still love that one.

Karen was a brilliant leader, the Chief Nursing Officer, and the life of the party. There was never a dull moment around Karen. I coached her one time to behave at a CHS national meeting. When she returned, she came in to my office sheepishly and confessed to a "dancing incident" whereby she might have embarrassed someone important to me at CHS. That was not the desired result of my coaching.

On a Monday morning, Karen walked into my office and was not in her normal happy mood as she needed to inform me of an incident over the weekend. A patient had arrived in the Emergency Department with some psychiatric issues requiring admission. Unfortunately, the staff had turned their backs for just a moment and the patient had slipped out the back door and eloped into the community against doctor's orders. We were legally obligated to hold the patient due to her condition so her leaving created a liability issue for the hospital. At the time, the weekend nursing supervisor was in charge of the entire hospital. She was one of the best with whom I had ever worked. But, that night she made a mistake and left the hospital to help the police find the eloped patient.

Karen was fuming and I asked her what she had said to the supervisor. Karen said, "I told her, 'you ain't Jesus!'" I could not stop laughing. Karen explained that the statement was an order that the supervisor's job is to look out for the many patients in the hospital, not the one patient that left. Of course, this was a reference to the Bible, Matthew 18:12-14. In Section 4 of this book I will explain how this led to forming one of my own Pearls of Wisdom.

I had spent twelve years with CHS and probably still have the record for continuous CEO tenure in the field. I was honored to have reported to David Miller during my tenure and he proved to be a fantastic mentor and boss. I used to tease him that there was only one thing that he was not good at doing – he could not seem to run me off.

I did eventually leave CHS when UAB Health System recruited me to return to my hometown of Birmingham, Alabama. I accepted the role as CEO of the system's 315 bed affiliated community hospital, Medical West. The hospital was in horrible condition and had suffered through a long period of strategic and operational issues. We were challenged not only financially but in terms of satisfaction and quality performance. I had difficulty finding any performance indicator that was trending in the right direction. Fortunately, and unfortunately, I never have backed down from a challenge.

I finally learned that there are some critical questions to ask during a job interview including how much cash the hospital has on hand. Two weeks into my tenure, I learned that the hospital only had enough cash to cover nineteen days of operations. In other words, we were basically surviving between bi-weekly paydays. As I had not asked this important question, I had walked into a major unexpected problem. As a result, there was no honeymoon in my new role and tough decisions had to be made immediately.

Three years later, that hospital had achieved a more than 400% improvement in cash on hand and had been profitable for all three years of my tenure, despite losing money eight of the nine previous years prior to my arrival. It was a nice run of profitability and for that I am proud. We also had managed to clear bond covenant defaults, refinanced our remaining debt, and borrowed another round of capital for renovations and new equipment. Unfortunately, I was badly bruised from the many tough but necessary decisions early in my tenure that had affected team, staff, and physician relations.

If you have wondered if I am an unusual magnet for crazy events in a hospital, I can assure you that is not the case. In fact, two of my favorite stories were experienced by my colleagues that also have served as hospital CEOs. The first story involved a prisoner who had been brought to the Emergency Department for care. The police officer that accompanied the prisoner and the hospital staff became distracted and the prisoner slipped out of the back door of the Emergency Department. When the police officer realized he had lost the patient, the officer ran into a back hallway and saw the prisoner shuffling down the hall. The prisoner was shuffling as he still had on his ankle and wrist restraints. The restraints were impeding a fast escape. The officer yelled for the patient to stop and the prisoner kept shuffling down the hall. The officer panicked and shot the prisoner in the leg. Twice. The prisoner ended up in surgery and I always wondered why the officer did not just jog to catch up to the prisoner and give the prisoner a push. The restraints would have worked much better than the bullets and likely avoided surgery.

The second story involved a construction project. The Facilities Director called my CEO friend and told him that he needed to see something they had found when digging a footer for a new addition to the hospital. The CEO viewed in disbelief what looked like human remains partially in the dirt. The police had arrived and quarantined the area. Then, the Coroner arrived. To make matters worse, a local newspaper reporter arrived. The CEO was starting to sweat. Just before the CEO called the system office in another state to set off the "Public Relations Alarm," the Facilities Director stopped him and asked him what day it was. Confused, the CEO said,

"Tuesday." The Facilities Director smiled. It was Tuesday, April 1, also known as April Fool's Day. The facilities team, the police, Coroner, and the reporter had all been in on the prank. Even though it was a carefully planned joke on the CEO, he was shaken by the thought that it could have been a real event. We still laugh about that story.

The stories above are really to explain that the life of a hospital CEO is full of surprises, chaos, and challenges. Most of those outside the c-suite do not see these challenges and therefore do not realize how tough leadership in a hospital can be day-to-day. One of my assistants told me that I had a switch I could flip and move from one dramatically challenging situation to another discussion while calm and not flinching. It was not unusual for individuals involved in the second discussion to not know of the stress and pressure I just had been feeling moments before.

Most healthcare executives face the same challenges and have a similar switch. What you need to remember is that when you are talking to an executive, you have no idea what is going on in his or her head. I encourage you to give them some grace if they seem distracted as they may be facing a challenge that has precedence over what you are wanting to discuss.

After 17 years of hospital CEO leadership in for-profit, not-for-profit, governmental, and religious organizations, I was ready for a change. I don't think I really "retired" from hospital leadership as I was 43 years old at the time. The Affordable Care Act, also known as Obamacare, was not a factor in leaving the c-suite as I actually was enjoying those challenges. A friend once told me I was sick for making statements like that. For the record, I strongly opposed Obamacare, then and now, as I did not see the model as sustainable. I did agree that the industry needed dramatic reform but I did not agree that Obamacare was the answer.

During my transition from the hospital c-suite, I had returned to the classroom to pursue a Doctor of Science Degree in Healthcare Administration, which I was conferred in 2015. That degree greatly transformed my approach to leadership and excellence in decision making. Before you ask, you do not have to call me Dr. McDougal - I reserve that for my students I teach at Samford University and for my daughter's boyfriends.

Now as a healthcare serial entrepreneur, I was determined to try to solve some of the problems I saw in the industry. Gylen Castle was originally formed as Leadership Underground to focus on leadership development primarily and offer a secondary service of healthcare sales strategy consulting. I had severely underestimated the demand for our healthcare sales strategy work and eighteen months later, leadership development consulting was discontinued. Today, we are Gylen Castle, a unique niche boutique advisory firm focused on effective and efficient healthcare sales strategy advisement.

You may be curious about the company name, Gylen Castle. As a McDougal, I have always been interested in our Scotch-Irish family heritage. Clan MacDougall fought alongside William Wallace for Scottish freedom and independence. Some of you may recall this war which was memorialized in the movie *Braveheart,* starring Mel Gibson as the hero leader, William Wallace. Towards the end of the conflict, Clan MacDougall had remained on the Scottish freedom side with William Wallace when England was cutting deals with many of the clan leaders. As a result, Clan MacDougall was on the loosing end of the deals cut with the Barons. I have pride in my forefathers' decision to choose freedom.

Gylen Castle is one of the remaining structures of Clan MacDougall and is a functional castle on the Isle of Kerrera. When my branding expert concluded we needed a new company name to reflect our pivoted services, I knew the name to choose and Gylen Castle, LLC was born. Gylen is properly pronounced as "gAH-lin" in the homeland but many Americans assume to pronounce it as "geye-lan" and I just roll with it either way.

My thought leadership with Gylen Castle is heavily influenced by my days as a hospital CEO. During my tenure at Parkway, Kathy was our amazing Chief Quality Officer. She is a spunky woman that calls it the way she sees it. She has earned that right as she is likely one of the best hospital quality experts in the country. One day, she appeared in the doorway of my office. She had a serious look on her face as she pointed at me and said, "Look here,

Big Boy!" Let's just leave it to say that she did not like one of my decisions and she was there to set me straight. I do not recall the exact topic that day as there were many times over six years that I heard that phrase from Kathy. Each time she said "Look here, Big Boy" to me it was intended to get my attention to *change my way of thinking.*

Over the past two decades, I have seen significant changes in the way that hospital and health system c-suites have functioned related to decision making. As a result, sales to healthcare organizations have become more challenging to navigate due to a very complex and long sales process to reach a closed deal. Healthcare decision making has pivoted to a new culture with new players and decision processes. Unfortunately, companies selling to healthcare organizations have adapted their strategies but not pivoted the strategies in response to the dramatic changes on the client side. Sales strategies have fallen behind in terms of efficiency and effectiveness.

You cannot out-hustle a bad sales strategy. You must think differently. You must pivot your strategy. Now that you understand my background and experiences, I turn our focus on the task at hand of improving your sales strategy to increase efficiency and close more deals.

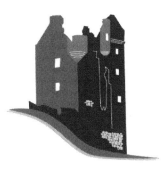

Chapter 2: So, What Changed in Healthcare Sales?

Hospitals are businesses. I have always been passionate about a hospital's operating mission focused on providing exceptional care to the body and minds of those in the community. The statement "no money, no mission" is also important. While at Baptist, Chuck called me one day and asked me to meet him at his car. I did not ask why and he didn't offer. I really did not need a reason. We headed to the airport where I had an amazing and unexpected opportunity. We were picking up a guest from the airport none other than Rick Scott, the legendary CEO of Columbia

Hospital Corporation. Rick was speaking at an event and Chuck had agreed to host his visit.

Chuck was an excellent leader and a strong believer that hospitals should be not-for-profit. Rick was a for-profit advocate, as would be expected. It did not take long for Chuck and Rick to begin the discussion of for-profit versus not-for-profit when Rick asked Chuck when he was going to sell the Baptist system to Columbia. Of course, this was said tongue-in-cheek. As a result of this question, I had the opportunity to watch the verbal tennis match. At one point, Rick turned around to me and said with a wink, "All hospitals are for-profit, or at least they should be." He was inferring that regardless of ownership structure, all hospitals must be in the business of making money. I never forgot that "Pearl of Wisdom" from Rick.

My entire career I have chased margin and profit. Before the healthcare altruism crowd gets too uptight with this, keep in mind that you cannot have a sustainable, strong margin unless you are producing high quality goods or services and you have satisfied patients. I was chasing profit but placing high value on the importance of balancing performance for all three areas of financial, satisfaction, and quality. If a company is weak in one area, the other two areas will suffer. For that reason, performance in all three areas are interconnected and for the hospital to reach its goals, all three areas must be improving in concert.

Sales in healthcare has become more difficult over the past decades. Many believe it is now just freakin' difficult. The reason for the increase in difficulty is the healthcare purchase decision process has changed. I have been in and around hospital c-suites for 25 years and the culture and environment have evolved. The result is a more complex decision process and a resulting longer sales cycle. Neither party want a longer more complex process. From my experiences, I believe there are four factors that have led to greater difficulty in decisions:

- The demise of the Cowboy;
- The rise of information overload;
- Increased competition for the decision maker's attention; and
- The emergence of the most dangerous person to sell to.

The Demise of the Cowboy. More than two decades ago when I entered the c-suite for the first time, there were a lot of "Cowboys" and "Cowgirls" running the show. I define Cowboys and Cowgirls as those who will go into the decision process boldly, often alone, and with little fear of consequences, professionally or personally. They are not afraid to make a tough decision even if they do not have full support from everyone around them. To clarify, they do seek support but they are not afraid to make a decision when the support is not there. They will also make a decision even when the data is not fully documented to support the decision. Cowboys and Cowgirls rely on data but also trust their gut instincts.

Moving forward, I will refer to both genders as "Cowboys" to make the reading a little easier. Some of the most aggressive and intelligent leaders I have witnessed are female so please pardon the sound of sexism as that is not intended.

I admired the Cowboys. I liked their boldness and willingness to take action. I also appreciated that they focused on the organization first and the greater good. Cowboys sought approval but were willing to go it alone if needed.

Today, there are still Cowboys but they are few and far between. The culture of healthcare has changed and the leaders have adapted. Many of the Cowboys have retired. The younger Gen-X and Gen-Y leaders tend to have a softer style where they are more meticulous in gathering data and, more importantly, gaining consensus. Accordingly, they rely on teams and other individuals to participate in the decision process. This is a direct result of a term commonly used at Gylen Castle known as Career Risk.

Career Risk is the perception of the leader as to how stable he or she feels in his or her current job. It is important to note that often the feeling, or perception, of stability is the defining factor rather than the actual stability. Career Risk is not a new concept in healthcare but it is now more prevalent in the c-suite. A decision maker that is feeling Career Risk will make perceived safer decisions to reduce their feeling of risk to his or her job and therefore career. Reducing risk is achieved through a variety of strategies including, but not limited to, selecting popular companies from which to purchase, gaining consensus from the stakeholders, and including others in the decision process. These strategies rarely include delegating authority for decisions but delegating portions of the decision process.

Standing and ad hoc committees are now meeting to discuss opportunities. Committees exist to increase more engagement of the stakeholders within the organization for recommendations and to have other leaders "own" some of the decisions. This is a good thing and it can be argued that the quality of decisions improves, but the process slows. In committees, champions must rise to carry a cause in these committees and if no champion emerges, the opportunity falls to the side. If a champion does emerge, the committee typically will make a recommendation for a decision and send it up the chain of command. Even then, there are times when the recommendation does not reach the decision maker. The reason for the loss of some recommendations is it is not just the decision maker that feels Career Risk.

Nearly everyone in the decision process feels some amount of Career Risk. A department manager may hesitate to make a recommendation to his or her boss if they do not believe the timing is right or the decision may not be viewed favorably. This slows the decision process as well.

For those reasons, the demise of the Cowboy has been a direct result of a changing generational culture and an attempt to mitigate perceived Career Risk. A strategy of delegation of responsibility for the recommendation portion of the decision to other individuals and committees has had a significant impact on the speed of decisions. But, the demise of the Cowboy was not the only cultural change in recent decades to affect decision making.

The Rise of Information Overload. Americans are bombarded with messages and information. Individuals are forced to intentionally, or subconsciously, sift through the information and try to retain what is important. This problem has grown exponentially over the past two decades.

Having more information is not all bad. We can argue information improves the decision process but the greatest impact is when a good opportunity falls to the side because it is lost in the noise. When this opportunity is not acted on by the decision maker, the decision was actually not to pursue the opportunity. As a hospital CEO, I realized that 95% of the time I would not commit to continue to listen to an opportunity after I heard the first brief pitch. This was due to the overwhelming number of opportunities that were presented to me. My sifting process was trying to evaluate a tiny piece of information regarding the opportunity, applying what I thought I knew about the opportunity and my organization, and then make a quick decision of whether it was worth pursuing.

Many of us are swift and make snap decisions. A typical website visit is less than one minute. A commercial on TV has to grab our attention in a few seconds or we divert our attention to something more interesting. Healthcare sales is no different. The impact of information overload has changed the way decision processes function in a hospital or health system. The executives are subconsciously sifting and without a strong Value Proposition Message, you do not gain the executive's attention. As a result, information overload is a major contributing factor to the pivot in decision making.

Other factors also affect the decision making process. One factor is competition for your opportunity. You may be surprised to learn that your competition is not just those you consider your direct competitors.

Competition for the Decision Maker's Attention. We have established that the decision processes have been intentionally, and unintentionally, evolving due to a change in decision culture and the information overload the executives are facing. We now turn our attention to the changes in the competition you face in the decision process.

Obviously, you need to understand who your competitors are in the sales process. When I mention competitors, you are likely to quickly focus on those companies that you consider to exist in your space in the market. These companies offer similar, if not identical, solutions and you compete to earn business from the same clients. From our high school economics training, we know that complements, or similar solutions, and substitutes, or alternative solutions, can shift the demand curve and serve as competitors to your solution. However, in a complex and long decision cycle, there are other competitors you must consider.

Your competition that is having the greatest impact on the healthcare decision process today are those challenges and related solutions that occupy the decision maker's attention and time. You could be in the compliance software-as-a-service industry subsector but if the decision maker is more concerned about an upcoming construction project, your competition for the decision maker's time are companies related to the construction project.

As previously mentioned, the decision maker is consciously working to improve financial, quality, and satisfaction performance. Success is the result of these areas performing in tandem and balanced. If one area is weak or declining, solutions to improve that area of performance will receive the higher amount of attention.

For example, if turnover times in an operating room suite between patient cases is a problem for the hospital, it is likely a problem for the leadership. Commonly this issue impacts all three areas of performance including financial, satisfaction, and quality. Obviously, inefficiency in turnover has a negative impact on financial performance. Quality outcomes are also proven to suffer when operations are inefficient. With financial and quality concerns, the turnover issue likely will receive attention. However, if a surgeon becomes frustrated with the turnover inefficiency, satisfaction becomes an issue. Now, the executive will place priority on resolving the inefficiency issue.

At that point, the decision maker is interested in any possible solution to improve efficiency, and therefore improve satisfaction. If your solution has nothing to do with this area of performance, your most concerning competition are solutions that do improve turnover efficiency between cases. To gain a decision, you must have the attention of the decision maker and competition for their time is a major factor that you cannot control. Self awareness of where you are in terms of importance to the decision maker obviously defines your competitive position.

This rise in competition for the decision makers' time most certainly impacts the decision process. This cultural change has increased in recent years and has some relationship to the demise of the Cowboy and information overload. In fact, the three prior factors have together contributed to a significant change in the culture of decision making. There is one additional cultural factor that is impacting the decision process and that person is dangerous to your ability to close deals.

The Most Dangerous Person to Sell to. There are dangerous people in hospitals and healthcare organizations threatening your ability to close a deal. You have likely sold to these individuals in the past but perhaps you were not aware of the danger you faced. I am not referring to some crazy person that is irrational and problematic due to their biases or lack of understanding. Rather, I am referring to a person that is not the decision maker in the organization but you need their support.

The most dangerous person to sell to is the person that has influence in the decision process and the ultimate decision but they lack authority to make the decision. In short, the most dangerous person is the one that can tell you "no" but not "yes."

In a hospital, this dangerous person is commonly a physician or department manager and you must sell to them. It is necessary. They are dangerous as they simply do not have the authority to approve the purchase but can have significant influence on the decision maker and affect the decision either negatively or positively.

You must sell to this person as the decision maker likely will listen to them. For example, the Facilities Director is commonly responsible for the building and its operation. They have a very important job and likely know the organization's facilities in great detail. You want to sell a lighting solution to improve their efficiency of power usage. You have a proven system and plenty of data. Unfortunately, the director is not convinced your solution makes sense for his or her organization.

There can be a variety of reasons for this doubt including he or she is just not motivated to implement the solution. It is possible that the director does not believe he or she has the manpower to implement. Or, he or she may be concerned about other issues that take priority over lighting efficiency. Unfortunately, you do not have access to the decision maker and the director gives you a "no" answer without ever consulting with the decision maker. This is an example of the most dangerous person to sell to in the decision process.

So, what do we do with the information overloaded, distracted, non-Cowboy decision maker? It is essential to understand that the healthcare executive is motivated. He or she wants to succeed personally and wants their organization to thrive. They do not want to ignore you any more than you want to be ignored.

At one organization where I was the CEO, I realized that opportunities were dying before they reached me. We were in a time of rapid growth. The team was chasing too many opportunities at once which was my fault and I realized I created a monster. The circumstances required this rapid change strategy, but that did not mean I liked it. I preferred a more methodical approach but we were forced to adapt our management style to the challenges that were urgent. My most precious resource was not money but time to implement opportunities.

As a result, my team was overwhelmed with work. If a team member already had too many projects on their plate, he or she did not want to add more. When a team member brought to me an opportunity I liked, I would assign back to that person the task of digging deeper and analyzing the opportunity. When the team realized this, they adapted and stopped mentioning opportunities to me as a survival strategy to manage their time. Many organizations are experiencing the same dynamics today.

When the need already exists for your solution, you are in a great position. The most critical step in sales is communicating or creating a need to implement your solution. If the hospital already recognizes the need, this step is completed for you. Otherwise, you have to create the need, and the urgency to act.

Most solutions have the opportunity to improve two or more of the areas of financial, quality, and satisfaction performance. The trick is to use an effective Value Proposition Message by *Selling to the Pain*.

The pain the hospital is experiencing is a problem area of performance that needs a solution to improve. Your success is based on your ability to identify this pain and propose a solution to resolve the pain. If the greatest concern is quality and your solution improves quality, focus on that aspect. By so doing, you can increase the attention of the decision maker and separate from the competition. The Decision Table helps to explain how this is achieved and then by applying the principles of Accountability Sales you have the opportunity to gain a favorable decision. *Selling to the Pain* is the strategy that pulls these elements together to close more deals.

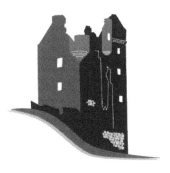

Chapter 3: Then, How the Heck Do I Sell?

An effective sales strategy is the key to success. If you have read this far, I doubt you question this point. Unfortunately, most sales strategies involve the typical method of identifying a lot of prospects and then working these prospects until a few become clients. This is an expensive and inefficient model for success, and sadly, very common. This is method is an inefficient sales strategy.

When sales are below expectations or projections, companies tend to use the "try harder" strategy. This occurs when companies continue to use their current strategy of working prospects to close but just add more resources. Company leaders add more sales professionals, spend more money on marketing, or even attend more trade shows. In other words, these companies use their same sales strategy but "try harder."

My advice is to stop using the "try harder" strategy. The truth is that you cannot out-hustle a mediocre and inefficient sales strategy. Rather, you need to pivot your sales strategy by *Selling to the Pain*.

You cannot out-hustle a mediocre and inefficient sales strategy. You need to pivot your sales strategy by Selling to the Pain.

Most of us are familiar with the sales funnel concept and while I am including it here, I do not plan to give it much attention as it has been addressed in so many books and articles. I mention it as it applies to our recommended sales strategy related to monitoring success.

The sales funnel is the concept of pouring potential prospects into the funnel and working those prospects until a few of them emerge as customers. During the process, they enter different stages including Lead to Prospect, Prospect to Opportunity, and then, finally, Opportunity to Client.

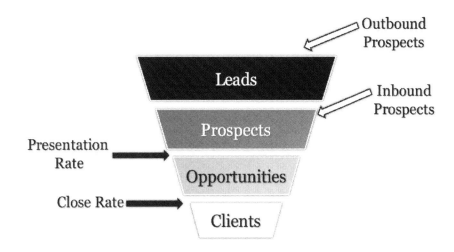

Most companies try to pour as many leads as possible into the funnel. When sales are not as expected, the answer of management is to pour more leads into the funnel in hopes of gaining more clients. This is the epitome of the "try-harder" strategy. Rather, you should focus on increasing close success rates for the prospects you are already gaining.

"Status quo, you know, is Latin for 'the mess we are in.'" - Ronald Reagan

Prospects emerge from two sources: inbound prospects contact you for interest in your solution while outbound prospects are those you reach through various marketing techniques to promote your solution. Inbound prospects are more likely to become a client as they initiated contact based on their known need. The cost to gain an inbound prospect is high as it is necessary that they find you and make the first decision to contact your company. Outbound prospects are less expensive as the advent of email and social media has improved this cost metric, but the close rates are generally lower. Regardless, obtaining prospects, inbound or outbound, costs money and time. Efficiency can be gained by converting more of these same prospects to clients. Don't try harder, but sell smarter.

Our strategy focuses on Value Proposition Messaging to work the same volume of inbound and outbound leads and convert more of these leads to clients. Your value proposition is essential to communicate to prospects how you can and will add value to their organization. In other words, you must communicate how your solution cures their pain. That is *Selling to the Pain*. The challenge is knowing when you are succeeding.

Measurement of your sales strategy effectiveness is often a forgotten step. I am commonly amazed that a company cannot succinctly explain how they measure sales success. You must know what is important to your success and measure the key performance points that drive success. Many companies choose to focus on Close Rate but measure this in varying ways. For example, some companies measure a Close Rate from cold lead to closed deal. Others measure from qualified lead to closed deal. There are many ways to measure close success but I recommend a two step process to reveal if your sales strategy is working.

Gylen Castle focuses on the two most important sales performance metrics of Presentation Rate and Close Rate. Presentation Rate is the percent of potential clients that you can move from Prospect to Opportunity. As suggested in the name, we recommend measuring to the point that you gain an audience for a presentation of your solution. Close Rate is also measured differently and we measure this as the percent of potential clients that you can move from the Opportunity stage to the Client stage. In other words, how many clients with whom you can close a deal following a presentation. We measure these rates in this manner as it takes skill to achieve consistent results with both metrics. We also recognize that success in one of the measurements can cause deceiving results in the other measurement.

Market forces can generate demand for your product or service and that may create a false sense of sales success. One client of Gylen Castle had a solution to address the pain of the ICD-10 implementation. ICD coding is a method established by the federal government for a hospital to categorize the care provided to a patient in a standard definition numeric code. Medicare and other insurance companies reimburse the hospital for care based on this code.

Hospitals were worried about managing the transition from ICD-9 to ICD-10 and fearful of a negative impact to their bottom line. There are approximately five-times the number of ICD-10 codes versus ICD-9 codes and that created a huge challenge for hospitals to determine the correct code efficiently and accurately.

As a result of the pending deadline for transition to ICD-10, 2014 and 2015 represented a time period when hospitals were looking for solutions to their "pain" to implement the new code set. This created what we refer to as inherent market demand as the customers were needing companies to provide solutions.

Inherent market demand for ICD-10 solutions created a false sense of sales strategy success for many companies. I have heard some tell me that the fear surrounding ICD-10 was similar to the Y2K fears leading up to January 1, 2000 when the change in date format from a two-digit year to a four-digit year for computers and other equipment. For the ICD-10 transition, the fear of lost revenue and rising costs were on the mind of hospital decision makers. This fear created demand for solutions and many companies with solutions were successful.

In October 2015, when the ICD-10 transition finally occurred without major impact to hospitals, companies that focused sales strategies to solve the pain of ICD-10 suddenly saw sales performance drop. In the year that followed, company leaders struggled as their previously successful sales strategies were not yielding results. What really changed was the loss of the inherent demand in the market. To avoid a false sense of strategy success due to the impact of inherent market demand, it is important to measure success appropriately.

As a hospital CEO, I experienced some years that had exceptional hospital performance. My first full year at Stabler, we had a 38% improvement in admissions compared to the prior year. Yes, that is an amazing year by anyone's standards. The hospital won a national growth award within our system as we surpassed every hospital in performance.

In that banner year, we were enjoying the benefit of a significant number of new physicians to our medical staff. We had also solved some problems for existing physicians that had experienced frustration with our admissions process. Our prior policies had created unnecessary paperwork for the physicians to admit patients and that led to artificial declines in admissions despite patients meeting admission criteria. For these reasons, I was able to explain our dramatic growth and I felt confident in our success.

The following year, the hospital experienced an unexpected decline in admissions. I spent a lot of time explaining the decline to prior year and writing action plans. As we studied the data more carefully, we realized that we had not given proper credit to a major factor in our 38% growth year success. While we had experienced some legitimate growth from our physician recruitment and changes in policies, what really put us over the top in admissions performance during the banner year was a horrible flu outbreak early in the year that was then followed later in the year by a bad gastrointestinal bug. Our success was partially due to some inherent market demand related to unusual community illnesses requiring admission.

If you fail to measure your sales strategy success using Presentation Rate and Close Rate as we recommend, you are at risk of experiencing a false sense of success due to inherent market demand.

Two years ago, while working with a client of Gylen Castle, I realized the power of success that results in performing well in both Presentation Rate and Close Rate metrics. The company provided staffing to hospitals. The contracts from clients were large and the margins were solid. From my assessment, it was evident that the sales costs were largely fixed as they had a stable and talented team that used technology and aggressive relationship building to add prospects into the sales funnel and close deals.

Prior to working with Gylen Castle, the company was doing well but they wanted to grow to the next level by significantly increasing their client base. They had a very high retention rate for clients so a new client was a big deal now and in the future.

Regarding sales performance metrics related to the levels of the funnel, each of the prior two years they would add approximately 300 prospects that resulted in 36 Opportunities and 6 new Clients. So, the Presentation Rate was 12% (36 Opportunities / 300 Prospects) and the Close Rate was 16.7% (6 Clients / 36 Opportunities). While performance was strong, the leadership was not satisfied as they desired to increase their Presentation Rate and their Close Rate while spending the same amount on sales resources. The results could be dramatic from improved sales strategy efficiency.

A year later following their implementation of the Gylen Castle strategy, the company had achieved a Presentation Rate of 18% and a Close Rate of 22%. That represented eleven new clients in one year, a significant increase from the six new clients in the previous year. The leadership team was excited as they were well on their way to reaching their growth goals as they had improved their sales efficiency.

To achieve these results, the company had shifted their sales strategy to *Selling to the Pain* by adopting principles of The Decision Table to better understand the decision process. Rather than starting by talking about how great a company they had, they now focused on the client and followed with assurance of their ability to deliver.

The efficiency was achieved by improving the company's Value Proposition Message so that their pitch was heard which resulted in a higher Presentation Rate. They also changed their presentation approach to focus on the challenges the potential client was facing and apply examples of how they had helped similar organizations. Finally, the company applied Accountability Sales hold the decision maker accountable for a favorable outcome. The result was a higher Close Rate.

The bottom line is this client learned the power of *Selling to the Pain*. The following chapters will unpack in detail The Decision Table and Accountability Sales to create an opportunity to understand why *Selling to the Pain* works.

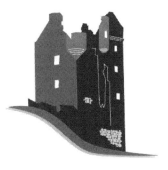

Section 2: Navigating the Decision Process

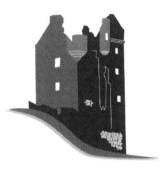

Chapter 4: The Decision Paradigm

In prior chapters, we have established the foundation for the next discussion of how decisions are made and the factors that affect those decisions. The factors are not necessarily what you think.

I have had a small number of seasoned sales professionals that share with me prior to training that they are experts in sales and are well beyond sales pitches. What they are nicely saying is they don't need my training. I heard this from a sales professional with one of our largest clients. I apologized if I had insulted her. I then asked her to explain to me what value her company created. She stumbled around for more than two minutes. My point was made.

Explaining what value your company creates is not easy and requires practice. Those that have pride in their abilities seem to struggle the most. These same individuals are often the ones that tackle me in the hall during breaks in our onsite training to retract their view of not needing training. One sales professional actually yelled to me down the hall, "I had no idea!"

Selling to the Pain is not sales training. Rather, it is a sales strategy. All executives and sales professionals have their own style for sales. Some core characteristics are important to success, including being likeable and organized, but most characteristics are unique to you. I do not desire to change your sales skill set but I do desire to encourage you to think differently. That is the intent of this book.

The Decision Table is our approach to explain how decisions are made. As an analogy, you do not have to know how a car works mechanically to drive it. But, you do need to know how the function of the car connects to the driver. This section focuses on understanding how decisions are made so you can apply your unique and effective sales skills to close the deal.

The Decision Table is an analogy in itself. I knew how decisions were made but prior to developing The Decision Table, but

I struggled with how to explain it. So, don't get too caught up in the analogy but focus on the factors that affect a decision.

Healthcare Executives are Crazy! If you have not actually said this phrase, you likely have thought it or heard it said. I actually once heard someone describe healthcare executives as "bat sh*t crazy." That was a little harsh, but the perception may not be that far off. It was funny to me because I was one of the crazies.

You may recall some of the stories I mentioned in Chapter 1 related to my days as a hospital CEO. That is a fraction of the stories that I have. The reality is the environment in which executives operate is crazy. They are constantly dealing with surprises, issues beyond their control, and many different stakeholder personalities. Further, I once heard someone say, "Management would be a lot easier if it wasn't for all the people." There is some truth there.

Most executives eventually become immune to two things: surprises, and feeling overwhelmed. The surprises are constant and never ending. I once thought that when I joined a new organization the surprises were more frequent early in my tenure. In reality, that was just my perception of the learning curve effect. For the first 18 months, learning the organization is a challenge as there are so many stakeholders and so many moving functional parts. It is also a challenge that the history of the organization is not known to you. The surprises are then thought to be due to lack of knowledge and understanding of the organization.

After 18 months, the executive typically has a moment where they suddenly think they know what is going on. At that point in time, something happens in the mind of the executive. Previously, the surprises, or challenges for that matter, were at least partially someone else's responsibility. But, after the moment, those surprises and challenges are now owned by the executive. Thus, the surprises seem to fade as the executive accepts responsibility for the known and unknown. They have become immune to surprises by accepting that they own the unknown.

Feeling overwhelmed is a constant battle regardless of tenure. From day one on the job, the executive is swarmed with challenges and opportunities and many struggle with forming a plan. In the words of Mike Tyson, "Everyone has a plan until they get punched in the face." The punches never end, inferring that the the challenges and opportunities only grow and start piling up. The executive's plan is then constantly changing.

"Everyone has a plan until they get punched in the face." - Mike Tyson

I was asked early in my career by a Board to create a five-year strategic plan for the hospital. I laughed. Out loud. I wish I could take that back but it was an honest reaction. An executive leads by establishing a vision for what the organization can become over a decade or more. That vision must be communicable, well thought out, and executable. The execution of the vision is the basis of the annual strategic plan. In reality, the one-year strategy plans we developed really only lasted 90 days before they were looking different. Changing market forces and the challenges and opportunities both internal and external cause the executive to shift mid-year. This was reality and further challenges the decision cycle.

Are executives crazy? No. Are their decisions sometimes crazy? They can appear to be crazy by those on the outside but they are never crazy to the decision maker. I recall a time when I announced I wanted to add a new cardiac catheterization lab (cath lab) at the hospital. I started sharing my plan and was actually called crazy. In reality, I had no intentions of putting in the new cath lab but our stakeholders were stuck in the mud on helping me come up with ideas for growth. We were complacent. My cath lab idea was to stir creativity. When one of the stakeholders told me I was crazy, I responded, "I may be crazy. But, help me find another way to put significant dollars to the bottom line by next year." The challenge was made and we had a great year of growth as the creativity was awakened by my "craziness." No, we did not put in the cath lab.

Is the decision process crazy? I would have to say yes. As evidenced earlier in this book, the environment surrounding the decision process is notably complex and terribly difficult to consistently navigate. By default, the decision process is considered by some to be crazy.

What is more crazy is that companies are not adjusting to the changes in the decision processes and developing a different and more effective sales strategy. The original mantra of Gylen Castle remains to this day:

"Insanity is knowing that what you're doing is completely idiotic, but still, somehow, you just can't stop it." - *Elizabeth Wurtzel*

Ms. Wurtzel is not the ideal role model. She had many deep rooted issues including significant drug abuse. But, her quote is profound. Many sales professionals and company leaders use the "try harder" method for sales growth. If they have a low Presentation Rate and/or Close Rate, they believe they need to add another sales professional to add more prospects into the Sales Funnel. Or, they need to spend more money on marketing. The issue of inefficiency with the "try harder" strategy created our core value:

You cannot out-hustle a mediocre sales strategy.

When I think someone has been acting crazy, I ask myself "What would a logical, rational, not bat-sh*t crazy person do?" Often I conclude that they would not do anything different. So, they are not crazy.

For that reason, crazy is a matter of perspective. When you stop assuming craziness as the explanation for behavior you do not understand, you can avoid using this as an excuse. A sales professional fails to close a deal and decides the executive is crazy. The executive chooses another company and he or she is crazy. The executive does not make a decision and he or she is crazy. No, they made a rational, logical decision to act, or decided not act at all. If you conclude they are just crazy you have chosen an excuse as to why you have not closed the deal. You also missed a learning opportunity to figure out how to succeed next time.

The executive is not crazy. In fact, most are highly intelligent or they would not be in the position that they sit. The decision process is really not crazy either. Rather, it is just difficult to navigate and that is why you need a method to understand how decisions are made.

The Sales Divide. You have a product or service to sell to a client. The Sales Divide is the deep void that exists between what you want and what the client wants. A favorable decision to purchase what you are selling bridges the divide and connects you to the client. The Sales Divide can be a source of frustration for many sales professionals. They take it personally at some level. As a business owner, I hate the phrase, "It's just business." When you are personally invested and passionate, it is more than just business. The Decision Table bridges the Sales Divide as you have an understanding of the reason for the divide and how decisions are made.

Almost daily, I read sales materials or talk to a company about their marketing materials. I am not a marketing expert nor will I ever be. I am a strategy expert. But, I scare marketing professionals as my approach to messaging makes them uncomfortable. We all have biases as to what strategies we believe will work. When I suggest sales strategies that are atypical of current marketing, the feelings of being uncomfortable rise.

I actually enjoy marketing professionals and welcome working with them. They have a skill set that has enormous value to organizations and I appreciate those that "get it." Unfortunately, a significant amount of marketing material is flawed as they are focused on extolling the virtues and values of your company. Truth be told, the executive really just wants to know you are capable, dependable, and a good choice. Other than that, they don't care. Testimonials are effective but the executive knows you are not going to share a bad testimonial.

Duct tape is a great resource for your sales professionals. If you want to know your prospects and clients, stop talking about you and your company. Duct tape is commonly silver in color. But, when properly applied to your mouth, it is gold.

Duct tape is not silver - it is gold when properly applied to your mouth.

Our Value Proposition Message approach is essential to success. If you want to close more deals, talk about the client and the pain they are experiencing in performance. The pain is what is causing the executive concern. You need to convince the decision maker that you understand their pain and that you have a solution to solve that pain. Then assure the client that choosing your company will not increase their Career Risk. In short, sell to the decision maker a solution that comes with peace of mind. To do that, you have to change your sales strategy to *Selling to the Pain*.

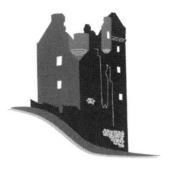

Chapter 5: The Decision Table

As previously mentioned, The Decision Table is an analogy to understand the factors of how decisions are ultimately made. The Decision Table has four legs. The first three legs include quality, financial, and satisfaction performance metrics of the prospective organization to which you want to sell. The fourth leg is the Career Risk perceived by the decision maker. All four legs impact the decision process related to what decisions are made and when the decision is made.

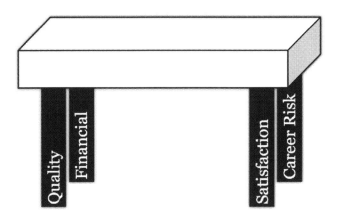

The four legs vary in length depending on their real, and sometimes perceived, strength of performance. A tall leg indicates stability and strength in that area and improves the strength of the table.

For financial, satisfaction, and quality performance, strong performance is desired and reflected as a tall leg of the table. For the Career Risk leg, when the decision maker perceives confidence in their stability in their position and career, the leg will be tall indicating that the feeling of Career Risk is low. In other words, the decision maker feels confident in their perception of low risk to their job or career related to decisions.

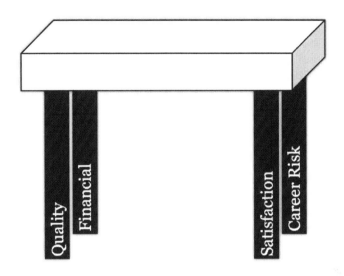

Strength of performance is important in all four areas equally. As you may recall regarding my discussion of "no money, no mission," I consistently strived to place equal importance on all three areas. If financial issues are plaguing the organization, it is very hard to focus on satisfaction improvement so ultimately satisfaction begins to decrease as a result to financial challenges. In those situations, I would personally feel more at risk.

To continue the analogy, the table legs are always rising or falling but rarely the same height for long. This can be due to actual changes in performance or due to changes in expectations for performance. The hospital could have had a very good year but the Board has expectations to improve more the following year. Suddenly, what was perceived as a tall table is no longer tall enough.

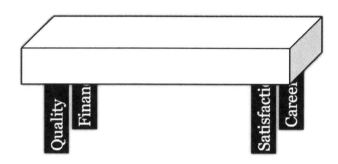

Obviously, an executive wants the legs to grow indicating improvement in financial, quality, and satisfaction metrics. And, they want to be stable and growing in their career which reduces Career Risk. To do that, they must make wise calculated decisions to achieve or maintain improvement and stability. It is a constant balancing act.

The top of the table is the place where all decisions are stacked. Every decision that could be made is placed on the table and removed when a decision is made. Keep in mind that no decision on an opportunity is still a decision of not to act.

Decisions can include strategy and operational opportunities from information technology, new revenue growth, employee benefits, new services, construction projects, satisfaction improvement, or quality improvement. These are depicted in the following image.

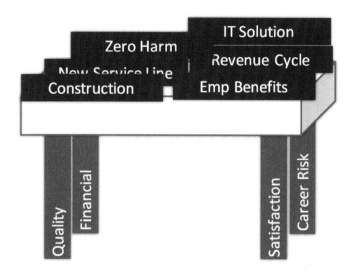

These decisions that are on the table are your competition. Capacity for decisions is really no different than resource capacity for operations and growth. Organizations have limited bandwidth to assess and implement changes to the organization. The key is for your product or service to have value that improves the organization in some way and, therefore, warrants a decision.

A stable table leads to more decisions being made. However, if an organization is struggling in one of these performance areas, that leg is shorter indicating weakness in performance. As a result, the table becomes unstable. When performance in one area is weak, a shorter leg creates instability and the organization is off balance, as an uneven table wobbles, and decisions become more difficult. Decisions that improve the area of performance pain for that weak leg begin to take priority and they are the only decisions that will remain on the table.

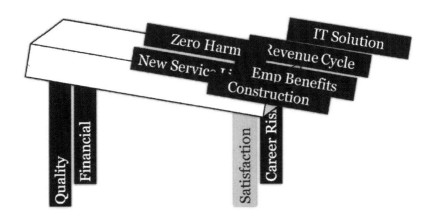

There are times when one of the performance areas of financial, satisfaction or quality declines, the leg becomes shorter, and the problem is perceived by the executive to put them personally at risk. You may recall the example of the turnover times in surgery. The satisfaction problem grew to a point that the executive started feeling Career Risk. When this occurs in two legs, the table collapses and decisions are simply not made unless the decision is essential to improve the weak performance area and the perception of Career Risk. The executive is essentially rebuilding a table by making a decision. But, they have limited time.

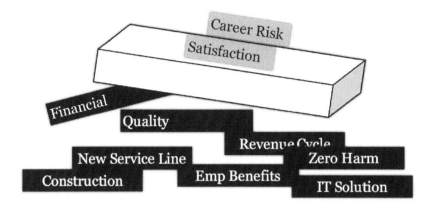

From this analogy we can now understand the process and factors of a decision. The mistake many companies make is to sell to the top of the table. As mentioned above regarding marketing materials, sales professionals misunderstand the decision process factors and focus on selling their company attributes.

Rather, these companies should be selling to the lower part of the table, or to improve performance of the legs. You may have a solution that improves financial performance and quality performance. If you are able to understand which of those areas of performance are weaker for an organization, you can focus your sales approach to that leg. That is our concept of *Selling to the Pain* where you adjust your sales pitch to how you can improve the area that is weak.

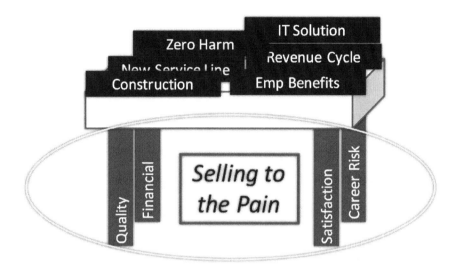

The challenge is to know which area of performance is weak, or in some cases, which areas of performance are weak. That returns us to our golden duct tape. When selling, I always start by trying to identify what is hurting for a decision maker. While some potential clients will be tight lipped and not share what pain they are experiencing, most are willing to share at some level. To find out, you use probing questions in a gentle approach. And, do your research.

Early in the days of Gylen Castle when talking to a prospective client, I jumped right into my canned pitch and got a quick "no." A year later in a conversation with that same client, I landed one of the biggest deals in our history. I was so close to blowing it a year earlier. In my early conversations with the prospective client, I did not listen to what pain they were experiencing. I was too busy selling sales development and in reality what they needed was a cultural change with their team. I did not listen first, and pitch second. The reason is I was selling to the top of the table, not the bottom legs of the table.

I have no formal training in sales and I have never held a sales job. However, as a hospital CEO, I realized that my job was to sell. I had to sell the present and the future of our organization to the stakeholders if I wanted them to help the organization reach its goals. I had to sell our next initiative on why it was important and that we could achieve it. In short, I believe leadership is sales.

As a healthcare entrepreneur, I must be a sales professional and I have learned the other side of the equation for healthcare sales related to some of my ventures. For that reason, I understand the process from both the perspective of the sales professional and the decision maker.

When preparing your pitch, do your research, bring your duct tape, and use The Decision Table to understand how decisions are made. Let's continue to explore *Selling to the Pain* with a deep dive into effective Value Proposition Messaging.

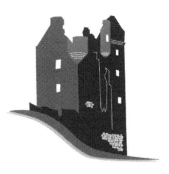

Chapter 6: Value Proposition Messaging

To sell effectively, you must have the ability to grab the attention of your audience and to succinctly explain the value you create. This value is communicated in your Value Proposition Message.

There are some individuals with marketing backgrounds that confuse the phrase "value proposition." Commonly, their definition is not a value proposition but a tag line. For example, Evernote's tag line is "Remember everything." I like it. For our purposes, the Value Proposition Message is totally different. It is a detailed explanation of how your organization and your solutions will create value for the client by solving their pain. The Value Proposition Message needs to include what you do, why it works, how it is proven, and why your company is the best capable to deliver the solution.

The Value Proposition is a sales professional's ability to demonstrate a working understanding of:

- The decision maker;
- The client goals and culture;
- The pain the executive and client organization are experiencing;
- The solution your company can offer to solve the pain; and
- Your company's ability to deliver successful implementation of your solution.

We will unpack these elements and then discuss the tools associated with effective Value Proposition Message communication.

The Executive Decision Maker. Large complex organizations have many dynamics in terms of how they are structured for decision making. For that reason, there are many players in the process. These individuals play an important role regardless of their amount of actual authority. We discussed previously the most dangerous person in an organization – the person that can tell you "no" but not "yes." Most of the players fall in this category. In fact, for most decisions there is only one or two people that can actually tell you "yes" with full authority, with the exception of very large organizations with defined delegated authority.

In hospitals, the primary players are typically Chief Executive Officer (CEO), Chief Operating Officer (COO), Chief Financial Officer (CFO), Chief Information Officer (CIO), Vice President, Assistant Administrator, Quality Officer, Supply Chain Manager, Risk Manager, and various clinical and non-clinical managers. From here, it gets complicated.

As there are so many influential players that lack authority related to the final decision to purchase, many sales professionals struggle with how to navigate the organization. Your point of entry is often not the decision maker so you must understand a variety of players that affect the decision process.

The reality is if you have seen one executive, you have seen one executive. They are all different in their roles and authority. This includes the CEO as their authority varies in different organizations. As a result, if you have seen one organization, you have seen one organization.

While every organization is unique, there are some tendencies among the players. The tendencies can be evaluated based on the size and ownership type of the organization. To unpack the influence of a particular player, our comparative points will include the following:

- Authority – the amount of authority in decision making the leader holds;
- Influence – who listens to the leader and how do they work with other leaders in the organization; and
- How They Roll – how the leader is influenced by others in the decision process.

If you can develop a general working knowledge to understand these three points when approaching a leader, you can improve your sales success. Keep in mind that these are generalities and we will all have the tendency to profile. But, profiling, albeit a dirty word in politics and political correctness, can be your friend.

For readability of this book, I will address only the CEO role in this chapter as the CEO typically holds a majority of the decision authority in a hospital. Other positions in the hospital that impact the decision process are addressed in Section 4, Pearl #5 if you are interested in my thoughts on those positions and the related characteristics.

Chief Executive Officer. For most organizations, the Chief Executive Officer (CEO) is the ultimate decision maker although they have limitations. As I shared, I spent 17 years as a hospital CEO in all different sizes and ownership types of hospitals. Most sales professionals do not realize how the CEO role, authority, and decision processes can vary between organizations.

As an example, when I was CEO of a for-profit hospital, my authority to sign a contract was limited to contracts that were no more than one year in term length and $5,000 to $20,000 in annual cost, depending on the hospital where I was serving. Yes, for many of you that will be a surprise. For any contract or purchase that exceeded those levels, I was required to gain approval from the corporate office. The impact on the decision progression was dramatic in that it complicated the process and slowed the purchase decision.

When I later became the CEO of a not-for-profit community hospital, I reported to a Board that had the ultimate authority for the organization. My delegated authority level to sign contracts jumped to unlimited term length and a maximum of $500,000 in total contract cost. This was very different from my prior for-profit experience. As a result of this significantly higher authority, you would expect that the decision process cycle was faster. In fact, I slowed my decision making because of the high amount of authority that I had and my perception of greater Career Risk. Previously, when on the for-profit side, I would make quick decisions and forward those to the corporate office for approval. Conversely, on the not-for-profit side, I would be very methodical in my decision making as I felt a lot more responsibility for each decision.

In terms of "How I Rolled," I found some of my Cowboy tendencies diminished over the years. This was partially the result of more trust in my teams and partially due to a changing set of cultural expectations for inclusion of others. I involved my team and committees more frequently to make recommendations prior to making a decision. I never ceded authority but I did listen a lot more to input.

I remember distinctly a meeting when I did not invite my team to join me to hear a sales pitch presentation. The company showed up with five members of their team to conduct the presentation. The company leader asked me if I planned to include my team. I found this offensive as I did not believe I needed help to understand the presentation. I don't recall if we did business with the company but the conversation did leave a lasting impression on me.

I was always ultimately a Cowboy despite changes in my authority and how I rolled. I made decisions quickly, boldly, and was comfortable without a lot of input, although I sought more input later in my career. But, as we discussed previously, I was a dying breed. Today's reality is CEOs are very interested in including others and conducting thorough assessments because they perceive greater Career Risk.

Regarding hospital ownership, CEOs in for-profit hospitals have less authority and face a longer decision process. This is also true for not-for-profit hospitals that have large system offices. In these structures, some of the decision making authority rests at the system offices.

Regarding hospital size, the smaller the hospital the more authority the CEO generally holds. This is most commonly true for not-for-profit hospitals. The smaller hospital CEOs also wear many hats and have smaller teams. As a result, smaller hospital CEOs are more likely to be Cowboys. I have operated hospitals from 52 beds to 315 beds, which had 170 to 1100 employees, respectively. From my experience, it is much harder to be a small hospital CEO. Some may assume the larger the hospital then the more talented the CEO. This is not necessarily the case as most CEOs I have worked with are equally talented despite the hospital size. However, small hospital CEOs tend to have a deeper working knowledge of the operations of the hospital as they have more direct involvement.

CEOs obviously represent the center of power in hospitals related to decision making authority. Even when approval from a Board or from the corporate office is required, the CEO still has immense control over what decisions are made and when. Understanding their authority and how they roll provides insight to you in closing deals.

Group Purchasing Organizations. The influence to the bottom line of a hospital for Group Purchasing Organizations (GPOs) can be substantial. However, I did not see a significant difference between the various GPOs related to cost savings performance. One of the colleagues from my doctorate program is writing his thesis on the impact of GPOs on hospital financial performance and comparing some of the GPOs. I am interested in what information he is able to uncover regarding the effect of participation.

When working with a GPO, there are two types of purchases including on-contract and off-contract purchases. On-contract purchases are those that buy from a GPO participating company vendor. Off-contract purchases are those made from a company that is not affiliated with the GPO. The influence of the GPO on purchasing decisions can vary from hospital to hospital. Generally, the influence depends on how much on-contract GPO purchasing is expected by either the corporate office or the c-suite. When working for CHS, we received a monthly comparative report of our on-contract purchases and this was motivating. I was more likely to buy off-contract with the organizations I led that were not part of CHS.

I also perceived an apparently significant correlation of on-contract purchases to the decision maker involvement in the GPO. If the hospital is part of a large system that has an ownership position with the GPO, then buying on-contract is certainly more of a priority. This also applied if someone in the c-suite has a committee or board role with the GPO but the hospital does not have an ownership interest. If a c-suite member is personally involved, the on-contract purchasing was more of a priority.

There are some industry changes whereby GPOs are increasingly more involved with services negotiated on-contract rather than the traditional products, equipment, and supplies. The most significant I have seen is the Parallon division with HealthTrust Purchasing Group. That division seems to be wielding some influence in purchasing decisions related to contract labor, consulting, and software technology purchases. That said, for most service companies, the GPO is not a major factor in the decision process.

Company Goals and Culture. Perhaps the most important factor in the decision process is related to the goals and culture of the company. If a hospital or health system is focused on improving coding compliance, and you have a solution for that need, you are likely to have more attention from the decision maker. Related to culture, if the organization is an early adopter of innovation solutions and you have an unusual new idea, the organization is more prone to purchase.

The challenge is to use available resources to study the organization and research what you can find. Related to Gylen Castle, if I sense a prospective client is complacent or happy with their current sales cycle performance based on internet research or discussions with leadership, most of the time the company is not interested in our services. I do not eliminate this client as a prospect but I don't push either by decreasing the frequency of contact and maintain a relationship. It is not unusual for our prospective clients to call us a year after we made the first contact. This delayed contact occurs as their needs have changed and they now are more interested in growing their revenue efficiently.

I highly recommend that you have a methodical process for assessing prospective clients. Gylen Castle completes a Prospective Client Profile on our leads. We study what we can find related to the company's structure, goals, and competitors. We also search for key words on the company's website that might indicate a desire for growth and a need for our unique solution. A key element we study is to determine the current value message the company is using and determine if we believe this approach will be effective. The profile also serves as a very valuable tool for if and when we have the opportunity to present our solutions in a discussion. We have found that as a result of our profiles, our Presentation Rate is much higher because we do a better job of identifying which companies to pursue; and, which companies not to pursue. We address this issue in the Target Client Definition section in the following chapter.

Assessing the current culture and goals of the company can also help you refine your message when presenting your solution. If you can identify early how your company can help the hospital reach their goals, you are much better positioned to close a deal. Your research into prospective clients not only improves your Close Rate but also your sales efficiency.

The foundation is established for understanding the players and factors that affect the decision process. Now, we move to *Selling to the Pain* as an applied strategy for success in sales efficiency.

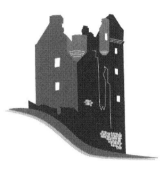

Chapter 7: Selling to the Pain

The key to a high Presentation Rate is your ability to anticipate and know the prospective client pain points. These are performance area metrics where they are struggling, or have concern, or feel urgency to address and improve. If you can discover this valuable information, *Selling to the Pain* provides an advantage to structure your pitch to focus on solving that issue of pain. This approach can differentiate you from your competition and can speed the close process.

Where is the pain? Generally, it falls in the four legs of the decision table – financial, quality, satisfaction, and Career Risk. It is not unusual for pain to be experienced in more than one area. This is the result of the previously explained interconnected performance for these four areas. In other words, if the hospital has quality performance issues, there are probably related financial or satisfaction issues that need to be addressed. Duct tape is a very effective method to find the pain – listen to the prospective customer for the pain points. While it is ideal to know the area with the most pain, sometimes you just have to assume and take a chance if the data is not there.

As a general rule, financial pain trumps satisfaction and quality pain. This is due to the fact that it is often expensive to correct satisfaction or quality performance issues. The financial performance area trumps the other performance areas in terms of importance to solve the pain.

Career Risk can also be a pain point. There are times that the decision maker just feels vulnerable and therefore feels at risk. This can be related to political or other pressures, internal or external to the organization. Career Risk issues are typically connected to another area of less than desired performance in financial, quality, or satisfaction metrics. A safe solution to fix the other performance area gives the decision maker confidence that performance will improve also leads to improvements in perceived Career Risk.

If your solution improves more than one area of performance in a meaningful and measurable way, choose the one that you believe matches the greatest pain felt by the organization. Once you have grabbed the attention of the decision maker with your solution, you will begin to build a foundation of selling peace of mind. Assure the decision maker your solution and company are capable, qualified, experienced, and dependable. With that assurance, you are better positioned to close the deal.

Selling to the Pain is a very effective method to design your pitch and presentation. Essentially, you are applying data to prove you have delivered value with prior clients.

Another critical step is to select your prospective clients wisely. Our strategy is all about efficiency. If you are wasting resources on those that do not have a need for what you are selling, your strategy is inefficient. For that reason, you need a clear definition of ideal target clients, and less than ideal target clients.

Target Client Definition. You must know which prospective clients are ideal for you. This is not only related to the structure of the client organization but their need for your solution, likely timeline to make a decision, and the potential margin for your company. I have a perfect example of why this is important. One of our clients expressed frustration related to Requests for Proposal (RFPs) from hospitals. A RFP is commonly a long series of structured questions and solution requirements that must be provided by a company to be considered by a hospital as a possible vendor. It is quite similar to an application for providing services. RFPs are commonly issued to a number of companies by a hospital or health system to complete a side-by-side comparison and serve as a negotiating tactic.

This particular company client of Gylen Castle was investing many hours in each RFP submission but realized that their Close Rate was lower than non-RFP potential clients. More disturbing, when they won an RFP and closed the deal, the margins were lower than non-RFP new clients. In short, the RFPs were a very inefficient sales process for this company. As a result of developing a better understanding of the impact of RFPs on the sales process, the company changed their approach on RFPs. Rather than chase every RFP opportunity, they became extremely selective. The new strategy they used was to try to break the RFP, or in other words, work with the hospital or health system outside the RFP process. For this company, the RFP submission process was all but abandoned. They have not regretted that decision and have grown their Close Rate and revenue.

While it is important for a company to know who their potential target clients are, it may be more important for the company to know those potential clients that are not ideal. Unfortunately, this is not common. Companies tend to take the approach of "don't turn away business." This is tricky. The key is to know where you are in terms of margin performance for the next deal. If a less than ideal new client will have a high gross margin, the deal may make sense. Or, if the opportunity is arguably a loss leader to create the opportunity for other services or clients that will have a desirable margin, the deal may be logical. If you are functioning inefficiently with current resources available, it may be advantageous to work with a less than ideal client. For healthy growth, new revenue added must be logical related to your margin goals.

I highly recommend that you consider a narrow definition of target clients and clearly define what organizations are not targets and why. This does not mean you have to turn down the business if they are not ideal but at least go in "eyes wide open" knowing you are straying from your desired client base.

The Problem-Solution Diamond. Once you have identified and understand the pain, it is time to build your solution to solve the pain. First, you need to understand what the client needs. They are searching for some combination of solutions to improve performance. They are also searching for peace of mind from confidence that they have made a good decision. Your handling of matching a solution to improve the pain will go a long way in earning trust and the business.

The Problem-Solution Diamond includes four steps that are interconnected. First, identify the problem as discussed above. Next, develop a solution and a plan to communicate the solution as a way to improve the pain. This was also described above.

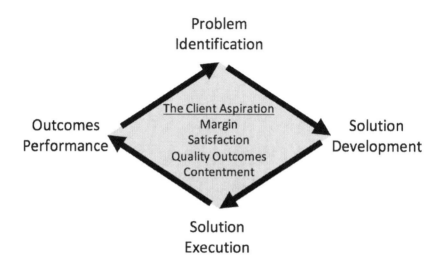

The third step is to implement the solution. In some cases, you handle the implementation for the client and in some cases they implement on their own. The best approach is to treat implementation as a shared responsibility with well defined roles. Even if the client is handling the implementation, stick your nose in there to assure a successful execution and support their actions. If you are responsible for implementation, assure the client is well informed of the schedule and update the status on pre-determined periodic timelines. A shared implementation is the best method.

The fourth step of outcomes performance measurement is essential and often overlooked. If you used an approach of *Selling to the Pain* and stated that you could improve performance, you have an obligation. You value the relationship with the client and you should care if your solution actually worked. To do this, you need data to track and monitor performance improvement. The client is normally excited about this unless it is sensitive or proprietary information. In that case, provide a template and let them track performance and ask for regular feedback to ensure their data is resulting in the desired improvement.

There is a side benefit to investing in data analysis as you have the opportunity to proactively identify other potential performance issues. When these issues have surfaced in your data but not realized by the client, you can help the organization avoid a problem. By proactively sharing the concern and a solution, you can endear yourself to the client. This must be done carefully so proceed with caution. Typically, I recommend an executive to handle this step to gain a closer relationship and sharing peer-to-peer is generally better received.

By using the Problem-Solution Diamond you have the implementation path for *Selling to the Pain*. At this point in our strategy discussion, you understand the decision process, the executives involved, and the elements needed to design and implement the Value Proposition Message. Now, we need the tools to communicate your Value Proposition Message.

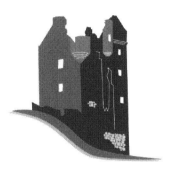

Chapter 8: Value Proposition Messaging Tools

The best strategy plans are worthless without inclusion of execution in the plan. The tools recommended to communicate your Value Proposition Message are the key to execution and include:

- 60-second Pitch
- One Pager
- Discussion Presentation

The tools are interconnected and build on each other to further expand the message of what value you create for the client and the trust the client can embrace in your ability to deliver. You should consider the tools as various ways to communicate your Value Proposition Message.

60-second Pitch. You may recall the story earlier in this book of the sales professional that thought a 60-second pitch was below them. If you feel the same way, get over it. Or at least call it something else to make yourself feel better. Regardless of what you call it, you must be able to explain quickly your company and the value you deliver to a client. Some argue that 60-seconds is too long. Regardless of the length, a well structured pitch in your own words will go a long way to gaining new business.

We recommend writing your 60-second Pitch to fully state your Value Proposition Message. By so doing, you have one document that serves two purposes. Generally, the 60-second Pitch includes the following elements:

- A gripping opening sentence to gain attention;
- How you solve pain that the prospective client is experiencing;
- A certification or case study from a reputable company that suggests you are qualified and experienced;
- An explanation of what the client should expect in improved performance; and
- Assurance that you can deliver your solution and provide peace of mind.

A Value Proposition Message of one of our clients is below to provide an example of an effective 60-second Pitch to communicate your Value Proposition Message. While this is a result from a client engagement, we have changed the name of the company and redacted a portion of the language. To frame this reference, the example company is a security compliance software and consulting company focused on providing assessment of security risk and problem mitigation.

Privacy security is often only a concern when there is an audit or breach. But, then it is too late to potentially avoid the audit or breach for your organization. At Red Rock Security, we can not only reduce your liability but increase your peace of mind.

Our XXX association endorsement is a reflection of our commitment to healthcare providers and our industry leading expertise. But, our raving clients are our biggest endorsement.

When you choose Red Rock Security to protect and strengthen your privacy and HIPAA compliance, you achieve many important objectives:

- *Expand Trust with Your Patients, Physicians, and Community;*
- *Reduce liability; and*
- *Gain Peace of Mind.*

Sure, there are other organizations that claim to improve your privacy compliance position. But, with Red Rock's advanced software we have a competitive advantage as you can:

- *Start Fast and Implement with Confidence without the Guesswork*
- *Reduce Your Worked Hours with our Advanced Automation or we can help you implement.*
- *Have the data at your fingertips when you need it with our intuitive dashboard interface.*

At Red Rock Security, we deliver Privacy Peace of Mind.

Unpacking the 60-second Pitch example will help us understand how this effectively communicates the Value Proposition Message to the potential client. First, notice the keywords identified in bold below. You may realize we are not talking about the company but the client. The client cares a lot more about their pain than how good you are.

***Privacy security** is often only a concern when there is an audit or breach. But, then it is **too late** to **potentially avoid the audit or breach for your organization.** At Red Rock Security, we can not only **reduce your liability** but increase your **peace of mind**.*

Our **XXX association endorsement** is a reflection of our **commitment** to healthcare providers and our industry leading **expertise**. But, our raving clients are our biggest endorsement.

When you choose Red Rock Security to **protect and strengthen your privacy and HIPAA compliance**, you achieve many important objectives:

- Expand **Trust** with Your Patients, Physicians, and Community;
- **Reduce liability;** and
- **Gain Peace of Mind.**

Sure, there are other organizations that **claim** to improve your privacy compliance position. But, with Red Rock's advanced software we have a **competitive advantage** as you can:

- **Start Fast and Implement with Confidence without the Guesswork**
- **Reduce Your Worked Hours with our Advanced Automation or we can help you implement.**
- **Have the data at your fingertips when you need it with our intuitive dashboard interface.**

At Red Rock Security, we deliver Privacy Peace of Mind.

Notice the keywords focus on what pain is solved, how the pain is solved, urgency for action, and the direct and indirect benefits to the client. We add enough information to build confidence in the company's ability to deliver but that is scattered throughout the pitch. Now, let's break down what we are trying to share with the potential client audience section by section.

Privacy security is often only a concern when there is an audit or breach. But, then it is too late to potentially avoid the audit or breach for your organization. At Red Rock Security, we can not only reduce your liability but increase your peace of mind.

In the opening paragraph above, we grab attention with an issue that the audience can relate to and understand. We also create a sense of urgency to act. Notice that the company is not mentioned until the third sentence and the emphasis is on what matters to the client, not how great the company is at delivering.

Our XXX association endorsement is a reflection of our commitment to healthcare providers and our industry leading expertise. But, our raving clients are our biggest endorsement.

Notice that we still have not talked about what the company does for the client. We name drop a reputable organization or draw attention to a coveted endorsement, as in this example. You can also reference an actual improvement for another similar organization to the client audience and what was accomplished for them. Finally, we suggest that while the endorsement is important, we are focused on the high satisfaction of our clients – that is what is important to the company.

When you choose Red Rock Security to protect and strengthen your privacy and HIPAA compliance, you achieve many important objectives:

- *Expand Trust with Your Patients, Physicians, and Community;*
- *Reduce liability; and*
- *Gain Peace of Mind.*

Now, we introduce what the company does more specifically but we are still focused on the client needs. The word "trust" is carefully chosen as a client would value having trust in a security company. Liability is a key point in that all organizations desire to reduce liability exposure. The objective here is to gain agreement from the client audience. They want what we are selling. Finally, we focus on the needs of the decision maker. While a strong relationship and reduced liability is what they want for their organization, we add that the company also delivers peace of mind to the decision maker.

Sure, there are other organizations that claim to improve your privacy compliance position. But, with Red Rock's advanced software we have a competitive advantage as you can:

- *Start Fast and Implement with Confidence without the Guesswork*
- *Reduce Your Worked Hours with our Advanced Automation or we can help you implement.*
- *Have the data at your fingertips when you need it with our intuitive dashboard interface.*

This final paragraph is key. We acknowledge that other companies provide similar services, but Red Rock Security is differentiated and better. We also finally explain that the company is a software-as-a-service company providing more insight. The three bullet points presented here were the result of studying the six problems the software-as-a-service solves for the clients. This list should not include two to four items to focus understanding. Again, notice the emphasis is on what the client wants and needs. We imply the capability and strong design of the company solution.

At Red Rock Security, we deliver Privacy Peace of Mind.

The above close is the most important part of the pitch message. Significant time should be dedicated to writing an effective closing. We want the client to remember the company name. As explained in previous sections, close with a personal note – we want to gain a champion that will carry our message through the difficult sales process. Finally, peace of mind is reinforced as a key value proposition.

At this point in the Value Proposition Message tool development, there are many unanswered questions about the company and how they deliver results. That is intentional as this is hopefully the beginning of an ongoing discussion. That is the goal. The 60-second pitch needs to lead to further communication including a One Pager.

One Pager. The One Pager is a well formatted sheet of information that expands the Value Proposition Message and adds more about what and how your company can deliver. Ideally, the One Pager is delivered in a follow up conversation to the 60-second

Pitch with a request to have a brief 30-minute meeting to further explore the needs of the potential client and the solutions your company can provide.

Development of a One Pager requires some time to create an effective piece. Generally, the One Pager should include the following:

- A restatement of the Value Proposition Message including the key words;
- A case study that shows how your solution has worked for a similar organization;
- Details about your company's qualifications, certifications, or other information that will give confidence to the audience of your experience and ability;
- A link to your website (your website should be an online brochure that is easily navigable to explain what you do, how you do it, and that it works); and
- Carefully chosen images to support and convey your key message points.

Do not overwhelm the reader with text narrative. A reader will read a limited amount of information so choose carefully what you include and select your images wisely. Charts and graphs can be effective to keep the attention of the reader. In the One Pager, your goal is to provide enough information to gain interest but we still have not shown all of our cards. Our sixteen-year-old son is still learning the art of "kiss the girl less than she wants." Leave the reader wanting more information about your value to his or her organization.

An example of the One Pager is not provided here as each document must be carefully tailored to your company and culture. Most importantly, your One Pager should expand on your Value Proposition Message and leave the audience believing you can deliver on your closing statement in the 60-Second Pitch. In our prior example, the closing was "At Red Rock Security, we deliver Privacy Peace of Mind."

There is singular goal of the One Pager to gain an opportunity to have a longer discussion with an audience for a presentation and discussion. That discussion is a presentation which I refer to as a Discussion Presentation.

Discussion Presentation. Once you have the commitment from your prospective client to listen to a presentation of your solution, you have crossed the Presentation Rate threshold. The goal of the Presentation Rate metric is to have a high transfer from brief pitch to a detailed discussion and presentation.

The Discussion Presentation is intended to be a PowerPoint supported conversation with the prospective client. The objective is to create a conversation but not to provide just a sales pitch. The meeting is not about your company but the prospective client's needs and how you can solve their pain. It is essential that the Discussion Presentation is designed to get the prospective client to talk about their pain. Once you know the pain, you can adjust your verbal part of the Discussion Presentation to focus on how you solve that pain.

Unfortunately, I cannot tell you how many times I have seen a company fight to get to the presentation and then blow it. When I was a hospital CEO and listening to various sales pitches, I personally had about a 5% Presentation Rate for companies that had delivered to me their 60-Second Pitch. In other words, for every twenty 60-Second Pitches that I heard, on average I agreed to listen to one Presentation. Thus, I had a 5% Presentation Rate, based on our previous definition, as a prospective client listening to a company's pitch.

When I did listen to a presentation, approximately 20% of the time I would decide to purchase. This decision was on occasion immediate and other times was delayed as we assessed the opportunity. Some companies view this as the close rate and 20% sounds pretty reasonable. From my perspective, it can be deceptive to measure in this regard if this is the only metric you are measuring. For example, using my personal example as a hospital CEO, I had a 5% Presentation Rate and a 20% Close Rate using our recommended calculation methods. The combined rate from pitch to close was a combination of these two metrics and a paltry 1%, calculated as a

20% close rate on the 5% of the pitches I listed to a presentation. That sounds depressing. My point is if you only focus on the 20% Close Rate, your company will miss the fact that your pitch rate, which we measure as a Presentation Rate, is very inefficient. Further, the overall success rate from Pitch to Close is very low.

The Discussion Presentation is essential to your ability to close deals. You have worked hard to get an audience and you want the potential client to purchase what you are selling. Unfortunately, many Discussion Presentations fail due to improper focus on things other than the client and their pain. Remember the duct tape? Stop talking about how great you are and use a presentation format to listen. An effective Discussion Presentation should follow this recommended format:

- Demonstrate an understanding, or probe deeply, to identify the pain the client is feeling;
- Express your understanding of the pain;
- Briefly present your solution to solve the pain;
- Explain for whom you have solved the pain in the past and name drop;
- Present the results from that solution implementation;
- Explain how you solve the pain;
- Differentiate your company from the competition;
- Justify that your company is dependable, experienced and will deliver; and

- Finally, create a sense of urgency with an explanation of how to get started solving the pain.

The above is covered in a maximum of 10-15 PowerPoint slides. The slides should be generic enough that you can adjust your presentation's verbal portion to address the pain point experienced by the client. Keep in mind that you may not know the pain walking into the presentation so this presentation requires some thinking-on-your-feet skill.

Regarding the actual PowerPoint design, use a very professional format and structure that avoids distraction. Carefully choose images that reinforce your point. Know your material so you can show a slide and talk about additional material. Also, avoid cute or "techy" transitions or distracting content so you can keep the focus of the audience on the message.

It is very important that the Discussion Presentation PowerPoint is consistent with the key words of the Value Proposition Message. This applies in terms of verbiage, images, and format. As a poor example of an attempt at a Discussion Presentation, a client of Gylen Castle provided to me their presentation as I was assessing their current strategy. This included a PowerPoint slide presentation and then a demo of their unique software that assisted with physician documentation in an electronic medical record. The concept of the company's software is to create efficiency for the physician and a more complete physician note in the electronic medical record. The company's presentation lasted 38 minutes including a 9-minute demo of the software. Unfortunately, I was not impressed.

The first 15 minutes of the presentation were about the company and not the client needs. When we reached the demo of the software, nine minutes does not sound like a long time. Unfortunately, a key point of the company value proposition was efficiency. Further, the company shared after the demo that a physician should be able to perform the same tasks in two minutes versus the nine-minute demo. For heaven's sake, if it takes 2 minutes to create a note in the software, show me a 2-minute demo. This confusing presentation caused me to doubt the capabilities of the software and therefore, the value proposition of efficiency.

This consistency of message also applies to the actual PowerPoint preparation. If your message is your company delivers excellence, make sure the PowerPoint is designed to support that value. A cheap looking PowerPoint will not suggest excellence. Further, on each slide you need to be pithy. You do not want the audience to be reading a lot of material and not listening to you speak. Remember that the goal is to address the pain the prospective client is experiencing and you may be thinking-on-your-feet with the verbal part of the presentation. This is *Selling to the Pain*.

You are making great progress. You have a Value Proposition Message and the related tools to deliver this message. It is now time to move to closing the deal.

Moving to Close. We have discussed at length the reason sales are so difficult in healthcare, how decisions are made, and a sales strategy to drive results. But, more than likely the decision maker has not said "yes" at this point. That is the critical leap that must be achieved.

Many times reaching the close is a waiting game. You cannot push too hard or you run the risk of offending the decision maker and losing the deal. But, what do you do when a decision has not been made and your frustration level is rising?

At Gylen Castle, we emphasize obtaining the decision to purchase that you desire. In the third section of this book, we focus on how to close the deal with a revolutionary strategy known as Accountability Sales whereby you hold the decision maker accountable to help you close the deal.

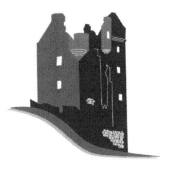

Section 3: Accountability Sales

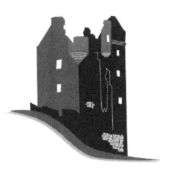

Chapter 9: My Sales Strategy Epiphany

As I shared previously, as a hospital CEO I was frustrated with the healthcare sales process and the time it took to close deals. And, I was the decision maker. It would have seemed more logical that the person selling to me would bear most of the frustration. That was not necessarily the case.

As we discussed in Section 2, the decision process is very complex in large organizations. The decision maker has many factors that are affecting their decision and the decision timeline. At this point in your application of *Selling to the Pain*, The Value Proposition

111

Message has been refined and the associated tools developed. You have presented your solution to the pain. But, a decision has not been made. You have not succeeded until you gain a favorable decision to purchase.

In late 2013, Gylen Castle had landed our first big name client of the GE Capital Healthcare Division. This was huge for our startup and quite intimidating. The training I provided included our insights related to The Decision Table and Value Proposition Sales presented to approximately 80 of their national and regional sales professionals. It went well. I had a clear understanding of how decisions are made in healthcare and the necessity to pivot the sales strategy to adjust to the decision culture. While I had a good understanding of the decision process, I did not have a good strategy on how to close the deal. I was missing a critical piece.

As I am research oriented, I started reading everything I could get my hands on regarding closing deals. There is a lot out there from solid strategies to crazy ideas of how to close deals. From complicated methods to cute approaches, there was a lot that was trendy, or even believed to be the proven methods, but not a lot that got me excited. I needed a credible and effective strategy to close deals that would match the healthcare sales and decision making culture.

I was searching for answers that would apply to the current challenges in healthcare but I was not finding them. As large as the healthcare industry is, and as important as it is to so many jobs and the very economic fabric of the country, I could not find any definitive work on the subject.

As part of my research, I had read the book *Crucial Accountability: Tools for Resolving Violated Expectations, Broken Commitments, and Bad Behavior (Patterson et al, 2013)*. A year later, I decided to participate in a training session. I admit that this was not a well thought out plan. I am a Fellow in the American College of Healthcare Executives and I had to obtain continuing education hours for re-certification. As the end of year deadline loomed, I chose a conference in Orlando, Florida. As I looked through the options for courses, one stood out at me as different – training associated with *Crucial Accountability*. I signed up.

The training was good and I learned a lot about how to handle difficult situations and manage through performance issues. *Crucial Accountability* is actually the third book in a series of work by Kerry Patterson, Joseph Grenny, Ron McMillan, Al Switzler, and David Maxfield (Patterson, et al, 2013). The overall premise of *Crucial Accountability* is that when another person is not performing as desired, you must carefully manage the communication to positively influence performance to expected results. This approach applies primarily when the gap in performance is important and relationships and associated emotions are at play.

I would venture to guess that 70% of individuals that read *Crucial Accountability* focus on application to personal relationships with the remaining 30% applying the concepts to work relationships. I believe that is due to the the fact that emotional issues we commonly face are typically personal rather than professional.

After the training and upon returning home, I was facing an issue related to our then 13-year-old son. I had asked him to accept responsibility to mow and edge the grass in our yard. Unfortunately, he was not doing a good job and I was having to remind him every week to mow the yard. He did not take the negative feedback well and when he forgot to mow, he did not like the reminders. When he had forgotten, the grass was then tall and difficult to mow. We were both frustrated. And, our close father-son relationship was taking a hit as there was tension neither of us wanted.

I then remembered a piece of the training in *Crucial Accountability* related to the Six Sources of Influence (Patterson, et al, 2013). I started considering the various contributing factors that might be affecting his performance. I did realize that I was now researching and analyzing an issue with a 13-year-old. Nonetheless, I had a problem to solve.

One day a few months later, I came home from work and the grass looked fantastic. I could not believe it. I found my son immediately and made a huge deal about his great performance and the fact that I had not reminded him. My quick praise had an impact. Rather than just be excited, I could not help but wonder why his performance had improved so much.

Over time, the praise was not having the same impact as initially. He was still doing a good job but his attitude was poor and I was now having to remind him to mow the grass. I had not solved the problem long term.

A few weeks later, our across the street neighbor commented on how nice our yard looked and asked me what yard mowing service I had changed to as he was considering a new service. I was puzzled until I realized that he did not know our son was mowing the yard. When I shared this information, he was so impressed. I had an idea to use this independent external praise to improve performance. I asked the neighbor to reinforce the praise the next time he saw my son.

I told my son that day what the neighbor had said about the yard and he smiled big. I was making some progress. Two days later, when the neighbor told our son his opinion, our son could not stop talking about it. A year later, we had the best looking yard in the neighborhood and our son was mowing on schedule and without complaint - well, for the most part as he was still a teenage boy. But, I had cracked the code to improve performance.

Shortly after resolving my "mowing crisis," I was struggling with a client that just did not seem to be willing to make a decision about an engagement with Gylen Castle. This prospect was a big opportunity for me and important to our growth. As I was leaving the house one morning, I was admiring our fresh cut grass and thinking with a smile that I wished this prospective client would perform as our son was performing. I am not suggesting that the client would mow my grass. But, I was considering how I could motivate the client to perform evidenced by closing the deal.

Unfortunately, the principles of *Crucial Accountability* are not effective related to sales strategy. In essence, *Crucial Accountability* is how to prepare yourself mentally for and to carry out a difficult conversation. If the issue is emotional and your relationship matters, you decide if the conversation is necessary. If it is necessary, you proceed through a process of understanding the gap in accountability. Once understood, you can express your concerns and hopefully change behavior (Patterson, et al, 2013).

At the core of understanding the gap, *Crucial Accountability* discussed the Six Sources of Influence (Patterson, et al, 2013). These are the influencing factors that are impacting expected performance.

	Motivation	Ability
Personal	Want To	Can Do
Social	Peer Pressure	Help From Others
Structural	Carrots and Sticks	Structure, Environment and Tools

(Patterson, et al, 2013)

To explain application of this table, when an expectation has been violated, the objective is to identify why it was violated. Another way of saying this is what factors are involved in someone not performing as expected.

There are three categories of factors including Personal, Social, and Structural as shown in the rows of the table. Personal are those within the person that has violated expectations. Social are those factors that are external to the person violating expectations but influencing the person's actions by either peer pressure or help needed.

Finally, Structural are those remaining factors that are neither inside the person or related to other people's influence (Patterson, et al, 2013).

These three categories are then separated into two types of influence including Motivation or Ability. Motivation is related to a person's desire to do something while Ability is whether or not they can perform. By combining the types and categories, there are six sources of influence that are possibly influencing the lack of performance. These Six Sources of Influence include:

- Personal Motivation – Want to – the person's desire to perform;
- Personal Ability – Can do – the person's ability and confidence to perform;
- Social Motivation – Peer Pressure – pressure from others that influences performance;
- Social Ability – Help from Others – the person needs assistance from others to perform and they cannot perform without this assistance;
- Structural Motivation – Carrots and Sticks – positive incentives and negative consequences that affect the motivation to perform; and
- Structural Ability – Structure, Environment and Tools – the availability of these elements so that the person can perform.

Related to our subconscious application of the above influences, most of us initially gravitate to assume lack of performance as a Personal Motivation issue. We assume the person just does not want to do as expected. In reality, it could be a Personal Ability issue if the person does not know how to perform. It could also be a Structural Ability issue if there are problems with the availability of tools necessary to perform the task. Once understood, you can properly address and correct the issue of performance.

Returning to the issues related to our son mowing the grass, once it was safe to ask, I probed for what changed for him. My first assumption was that the issue had been a Personal Motivation issue and that he just did not want to mow the grass, much less do a good job. I then thought that perhaps he had some peer pressure from friends that it was not cool to do good work for your dad.

When asked, my son responded that the issue had been lack of confidence in his ability to perform. He knew how to push a lawn mower but, he did not feel confidence in how to use the equipment and the techniques in performing the task. I was trying to fix what I thought was a Personal Motivation issue and I had been wrong. The issues were Personal Ability as he did not think he knew the techniques or how to properly use the equipment to do a good job. My improper assessment led to a longer process to correct performance.

I had evidence that the Six Sources of Influence could improve performance related to tasks on a personal level. But, I was struggling to use this method on a professional level as a strategy to close deals. I admit that at this point I hit a wall related to applying

Crucial Accountability to sales strategy. At the heart of the conflict in application was that *Crucial Accountability* has a cornerstone of an emotional connection between the parties. That is not the case in sales. I needed to get out of the box to develop a new strategy.

The problem in performance I was facing was when a prospective client did not make a decision or did not make the decision that I desired. I believed that I needed to hold this person accountable to help me close the deal. I paused because that was potentially outrageous and so far outside the norm of expectations. Who was I to think that I could, or should, hold a decision maker accountable?

But, was it outrageous? We hold friends, family, coworkers, subordinates, and even our supervisors accountable to perform. We also hold ourselves accountable to perform. So, was it outrageous that we would hold prospective clients accountable to help us close a deal? I reached the conclusion that this was different but not outrageous. I began down a path of the radical new concept of Accountability Sales.

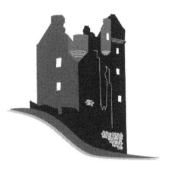

Chapter 10: Accountability Sales Confluence

The result of my work was the development of the Accountability Sales Confluence. A confluence is when two objects come together to form one object. An example is two streams that merge to form a river. I needed the desires of the prospective client and my desires to come together if I wanted to close deals. The below table is how the generic framework of Accountability Sales Confluence functions. While there are some similarities to the Six Sources of Influence in *Crucial Accountability* (Patterson, et al, 2013), these similarities other than structure quickly fade when moving to application. Keep in mind that we are focused on the performance of the decision maker in the organization to whom we are selling.

	Motivation	**Ability**
Internal	Is the Decision Maker not motivated?	Does the Decision Maker have authority?
People	Does the Decision Maker require help or cover?	What person(s) are needed to help make a decision?
External	Is the Decision Maker dealing with competing demands?	What resources are needed?

The aligning of Motivation and Ability with Internal, People, and External attributes creates six factors that could be affecting the performance of the decision maker. Each factor is different and therefore requires a different approach to resolving the lack of performance.

- Internal Motivation – Lack of Motivation - the decision maker simply does not have the motivation to close the deal.

- Internal Ability – Lack of Ability – the decision maker does not know how, have the necessary authority, or have sufficient confidence to close the deal.

- People Motivation – Requires Cover – the decision maker feels pressure from others to choose another alternative or not close the deal.
- People Ability – Assistance from Others – the decision maker needs others to help close the deal.
- External Motivation – Incentives – the decision maker has incentives that are conflicting with closing the deal.
- External Ability – Needed Resources – the decision maker may not have the resources to close the deal.

To understand the differences in the above factors, examples are helpful. Internal Ability could be related to the contract terms exceeding the authority of the decision maker. People Motivation could be when there is disagreement among a committee as to which company should be chosen for a solution and the decision maker does not want the conflict of a decision without consensus.

People Ability could be that the decision maker has delegated some of the decision process to a committee and the committee has not, or will not, act to make a recommendation. External Motivation may be related to the decision maker having a year end performance evaluation upcoming and other decisions are taking precedence over the decision you desire. Finally, External Ability could be a lack of IT department resources allocated to implement a technology solution you have proposed.

Clearly, the differences in the above circumstances would require a different approach to resolve the issue. As the situations differ, your strategy to hold the decision maker accountable is also different. In the next chapter, we explore how to apply Accountability Sales to navigate a decision process and to hold the decision maker accountable to help you close the deal.

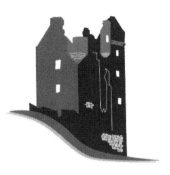

Chapter 11: Accountability Sales

With the Accountability Sales strategy, we have a way to unpack the issue of performance related to closing the deal by holding the decision maker accountable. The Confluence is an element of the larger strategy. To properly close a deal, I recommend using our six steps to Accountability Sales.

Each of these steps requires significant preparation and implementation on your part to close the deal. We will explore each step in detail with the objective to increase your Close Rate.

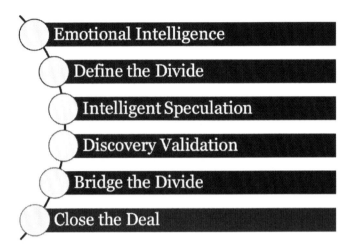

Emotional Intelligence - It's them, not you. Ok, maybe it is you. The first step is to prepare yourself to navigate the process and close the deal. In Section 2 of this book, we developed the concept of the Value Proposition Message and noted the importance of your messaging tools. In this Chapter, we focus on preparing yourself to deliver the message and manage the Accountability Sales framework. Specifically, this chapter focuses on the Emotional Intelligence step in the framework.

"I think the worst enemy to success is our anxiousness to get it." - *Antonio Banderas*

We often are our own worst enemy in the close process. We push too hard. We make too many assumptions. We assume that if it makes sense to us then it makes sense to everyone else. I have been the very victim of my own overconfidence. Just because "I get it" does not mean anyone else "gets it." When in that situation, you don't close many deals.

You need to look internal and take an inventory of what attributes you possess that suggest you are truly good at sales. My success has been related to my ability to listen to the client and then adjusting my pitch and message to their needs. In other words, I am pretty good at thinking-on-my-feet. If you can develop a belief by the client that you have a solution to their pain, you have taken a large step towards closing the deal.

The reality is to be good at sales you have to design an effective Value Proposition Message, prepare yourself to present the message, and then navigate a framework to achieve closed deals. We have our message path. Now, let's work on ourselves.

In 2012, the University of Alabama softball team won its first national championship. I am an out-of-the-closet college softball fan. I find the in-game strategy fascinating and the energy of the players contagious. Sales professionals should be no different in regard to excitement related to their next pitch. You hope that excitement is contagious to the prospective client.

During the 2012 College Softball World Series, one of the television commentators held up a book that was said to be a springboard for the year of success for the University of Alabama softball team. The book referenced was *Bricks, Fish Hooks, Toilets and Pride* by Brian Cain (2011). That actually is the name of the book; and, yes, I read it. The book is built around sports psychology concepts that you must prepare yourself mentally for the next pitch, or play, or sports activity, and then you have greater opportunity for success.

While the book does not address sales strategy, I found the application of one principle very useful. At the core of Cain's philosophy is the equation E+R=O, or Event + Response = Outcome (Cain, 2011). There are very few events that happen around us that we can control. However, we have total control of our responses to the events. The combination of the event plus our response results in the outcome (Cain, 2011). This philosophy supports that we should not focus on an event but focus on our response to the event.

For example, if we do not receive a favorable response to our 60-Second Pitch and gain a presentation opportunity, we cannot control that event. We can control our response to the unfavorable decision. Last year, a client nicely told me they did not need the services of Gylen Castle. The message I received was shortsighted. I had researched the company and I knew their current approach to solving a pain in the industry was fading in effectiveness due to changing market needs. I could have responded with data or client testimonials to prove the client needed us or argued with their overconfidence in their current approach. Rather, I controlled my response and told the client I understood and I was excited about their past and their confidence in future success. I also maintained a relationship that became more collegial rather than sales oriented as the CEO and I talked periodically about management strategy. Six months after being told we were not needed, I landed the contract for the same services I had pitched earlier. My control of my response to an unfavorable event led to an eventual favorable outcome.

As stated previously, the key to performance success in sales is to focus on what matters which is closing deals. Many of us are trapped in believing that we are really good at sales because of our ability to build relationships. In reality, what matters is our ability to close deals. We must focus on that metric of performance. Tony Dungy had great success as a head coach with the NFL franchise Indianapolis Colts and he credited his success to his ability to focus the players on what matters, winning games. The players could not fear failure or losing the game. They also could not focus on things that did not lead to winning games. Rather, they had to focus on what they could control and that was their performance on the next play.

"Don't fear failure. Fear being successful at things that don't matter." - Tony Dungy

The other challenge we need to guard against what I refer to as "half emotions" related to when we overreact in one of two ways. First, we fail to prepare our research or we believe we know more than we really do and the result is to go in "half informed." When we assume we know more than our prospective client, we are doomed. Rather, assume you know little and you can learn a lot. Remember to apply the gold duct tape.

The other "half emotion" is to go in "half cocked." Most sales professionals are emotional people and have their share of confidence. I think that is just part of the job and a side effect of other necessary personality traits. Emotions can take you a long way on the road to success but misplaced emotions can be a killer. I have the 24-hour rule. When I hear or read something that causes my negative emotions to rise, I pause for 24 hours before responding. These emotions include frustration, anger, or disappointment. I cannot always wait the 24 hours but I have been surprised how often I can wait. The 24 hours gives me some time to prepare my response and to allow the emotions to fade. By carefully planning our responses to events and managing our "half emotions" we have the opportunity to close more deals. Self awareness is a great place to start.

Another danger in preparation is stacked assumptions. One assumption that is not supported by fact or data can be dangerous. Stacking multiple unverified assumptions can leave you ill prepared to close the deal. An example is you assume that the decision maker believes your solution is consistent with their goals for the year. Then, you assume that there is a sense of urgency to implement the solution. Next, you assume the contract should be signed in the next 30 days. Your stacked assumptions have created an unrealistic internal expectation that is supported only by your opinions and not facts. When the decision maker fails to meet your falsely developed expectations, you run the risk of responding emotionally and potentially blowing the deal.

You have worked very diligently to prepare your pitch. You must work just as hard on preparing your internal skills to effectively manage the close process. For that reason, we can create our own formula P+EC=CD, or Preparation + Emotional Control = Closed Deals.

Now that you are prepared externally with your Value Proposition Message tools and prepared internally through emotional intelligence, you are ready to move to the next step of Define the Divide.

Define the Divide. To begin with unpacking the decision, we must know what is the divide, or issue with which we are dealing. In most cases related to this book, the divide is related to a lack of the decision we desire. This can be in two forms. First, the decision maker has made, or we believe they will make, a decision that is unfavorable to our goal of closing the business deal. This could be choosing another competing company for the solution. The second form of divide is when a decision has not been made. To think about this differently, a decision has actually been made as the decision maker has decided not to decide now. It is ok to re-read that sentence.

At this point, you believe you have a divide but the challenge is to choose the right course of action. You also face a decision of should you take action by trying to advance the decision or allow the decision process to continue without your intervention.

Consider the previous quote by Antonio Banderas, "I think the worst enemy to success is our anxiousness to get it." If you are a dedicated and passionate sales professional, a sense of urgency is likely part of your DNA. Yes, you want it now. You are likely competitive and determined.

If you are anything like me, you prefer a mantra of "Anything worth doing was worth doing yesterday." I hate waiting. If I have made a decision and do my part, I think the other person should do the same. I prefer to cross the finish line on this task or sale and move to the next challenge. Unfortunately, pushing a decision maker to take action could harm my ability to close the deal. When facing this divide, you must pause to answer three critical questions before you decide to take action:

1. Does it really matter if the decision maker decides now?
2. Does the decision maker feel a sense of urgency?

3. What are the advantages and dangers of pushing a decision?

First, we must answer if it is critical for a decision to be made now. I want it done now for the reasons described above. But, does it really matter? The answer could be it does matter but make sure there are valid reasons for you and the decision maker that now is the right time. Some of the best deals are closed when the issue is not forced.

The second question is related to the decision maker's sense of urgency. You likely feel a sense of urgency or you would not see a divide in performance. The decision maker's sense of urgency is the real issue here. Action on your part to bridge the divide could backfire and harm your chances of closing the deal if shared urgency does not exist. If you decide that the decision maker does not feel a sense of urgency, this is a challenge for you. You must ask yourself if there is risk to the decision maker as a result of delays. If the risk is low, you should likely pause when considering addressing the divide. But, if the risk is high, you need a new strategy to communicate the risks in a manner that is motivating.

I have experienced this personally. I would push for a decision and make regular contact with prospective clients typically on a weekly basis. I was smart that I did not push hard and I would mix in verbal and written contact, and even sometimes use a news article of mutual interest to make contact. As Gylen Castle grew, I did not have as much time for follow up with prospective clients and the contact intervals increased to three to four weeks between each contact. Interestingly, my Close Rates improved and the time required to close deals was not any longer than before.

The third question is an internal honest assessment – if I push for action, what are the risks of pushing? This is a calculated risk benefit analysis as if the risks outweigh the benefits, you have a divide that is not worth pushing for the decision maker to take action.

Answering the above three questions will validate if you need to bridge the divide now. If you determine the divide is not as monumental as you perceived, it is best to wait. However, if you believe the answers to these three questions justifies that you take action to influence a decision maker, you have a divide that needs to be addressed. The challenge is how to do this. If you believe intervention and action is necessary and appropriate to advance to close the deal, you are ready to develop your strategy for action.

As we work through the steps of Accountability Sales, an example will be a useful approach. You are selling a training service to a hospital to support their implementation of a new Electronic Medical Record (EMR). The purpose of the EMR is to capture and manage all patient information in a complex software. Cerner is the EMR company and they do not provide training for go-live implementation of their software for your physicians, nurses, and staff. For that reason, the hospital needs to select a training and implementation consulting company to provide this training service. Your company typically provides 25-300 training consultants onsite at the hospital, depending on the size of the hospital, to train and assist the hospital staff with learning the new Cerner EMR system.

The hospital has relied on a team to evaluate the five companies. While the CEO has retained decision authority, the COO is tasked with receiving a recommendation from the team and then subsequently making a recommendation to the CEO. Your company is on the "short list" of five companies for the contract and you provide a Discussion Presentation to the COO and the team.

Following the presentations, you are told that your company is in the final three. Your competitors include the largest EMR training company in the country, and a company that provided training for a sister hospital in the same large hospital system two years ago. You have the smallest company of the three "finalists" and you compete on excellence, hands-on management, high satisfaction, and you are significantly lower in cost than the other finalists.

Selecting a training company is a potentially risky decision for the hospital. Specifically, you know that a poor go-live implementation could have near-term and long-term financial, quality, satisfaction, and Career Risk implications. Such risks of a poor or ineffective implementation by the hospital include:

- The EMR is not used to its potential not only now but in the long run having lasting effects;
- The large investment in the benefits of Cerner could be reduced in value to the hospital;
- Physician and nurse satisfaction could suffer if they are not happy with the performance of the EMR training company selected and could lead to turnover;
- Physicians could become frustrated and move referred services to other hospitals as the EMR is perceived as difficult to use (I actually watched from a distance an unofficial surgeon 30-day strike related to a poor EPIC EMR implementation);
- The hospital may have to invest in additional and unanticipated follow up training costing thousands of dollars and countless wasted man-hours; and
- The decision maker could have a "black eye" from selecting the wrong company (In fact, I have seen CEOs lose jobs when an EMR implementation goes poorly).

Accordingly, the risks to the hospital and the decision maker are real which can lead to a treacherous decision process. Following notification that you are a finalist, the hospital informs you that a decision will be made in three weeks, on or before August 1, for an October 15 go-live.

Unfortunately, it is now August 15 and no decision has been made. To add to the challenges of no decision, you know that lining up the consulting resources for the training with less than 60 days notice is a big challenge. For that reason, you are feeling anxious and wonder if you need to take action to try to help advance the decision process.

As previously explained, the first step is to Define the Divide. In the above example, the divide is inaction by the hospital to select one of the three finalist companies to provide the training services. More specifically, the divide is that your company has not been chosen.

You then answer the three questions posed previously:

1. Does it really matter if the decision maker decides now?
    Yes, the hospital imposed timeline not only could increase your costs but put at risk your ability to deliver a high quality and satisfaction service. You really need an answer in the next seven days.
2. Does the decision maker feel a sense of urgency?
    Yes, or at least they should, based on the hospital determined schedule for go-live.
3. What are the advantages and dangers of pushing a decision?
    A decision soon is advantageous for both the hospital and the company selected. The danger to your company is

being perceived as "pushy" related to the decision and that could harm your ability to close the deal.

From the answers to the above questions, you conclude that it is appropriate for you to initiate action to try to advance the decision process of selecting a training company. You also believe that due to your competition, a more proactive approach would be beneficial. The next step is to use Intelligent Speculation to determine the factor, or factors, affecting the lack of the decision. By so doing, you can form a plan to take action to cross the divide to a decision.

Intelligent Speculation*.* This step is important but tricky to navigate. We have determined there is a divide that needs action on our part to move towards closing the deal. The challenge is to determine the best strategy to take action to hold the decision maker accountable to close the deal.

The approach recommended is the scientific method of establishing a hypothesis and then testing the hypothesis for validation. The testing process is not to reach 100% confidence but 90% confidence. We recommend a 10% threshold of significance, similar to statistical testing at a level of two deviations from the mean. My statistics professors would be proud of me but you are probably yawning. So, let's simplify the concept. Using the scientific method, you are determining what you believe the issue is that is causing the divide (hypothesis) and then working through steps to determine if you have confidence that you are 90% correct (testing significance).

This is the step where we apply the Accountability Sales Convergence matrix. There are six possible factors that may be causing the divide. The challenge is to determine which factor is contributing to the divide so that we can form a plan to help address and resolve the divide to close the deal.

	Motivation	Ability
Internal	Is the Decision Maker not motivated?	Does the Decision Maker have authority?
People	Does the Decision Maker require help or cover?	What person(s) are needed to help make a decision?
External	Is the Decision Maker dealing with competing demands?	What resources are needed?

Selecting one of the six factors is a challenge and the risk of taking action based on selection of the wrong factor can be a deal killer. For that reason, it is necessary to proceed with caution.

To effectively use the Confluence Matrix, I recommend three steps. First, begin with a negation approach where you will eliminate 50% of the factors. This is basically deciding what factors are not at play. The second step is to narrow the three remaining possible factors to two factors. And, the final step is to choose one factor that will become the center of our hypothesis of the cause of the divide but we will keep in mind that the second factor could also be the contributing factor.

Let's return to our example and apply the Confluence Matrix. The first of three steps is to eliminate three of the factors. Due to the likely priority of effective implementation of the EMR, you eliminate both External factors. Related to External Ability, higher priority competing demands for resources are unlikely due to the looming implementation deadline. Due to the risks of a poor implementation, the incentives should be aligned for action which eliminates External Motivation as a factor.

You also remove Internal Motivation as a factor as there is no reason to believe that the decision maker lacks motivation. We believe this to be true as we know the Cerner implementation is a priority for the hospital and the decision maker would not likely lack motivation to make a decision by the deadline.

Next, we move to step two of using the Confluence Matrix to narrow from the remaining three factors to two. The three remaining factors include: Internal Ability, People Motivation, and People Ability. The second step requires more boldness to eliminate one of the remaining factors as you are moving towards forming your hypothesis.

You begin with evaluating the factor of Internal Ability of the decision maker which is related to the authority to act. Due to the importance of the project, it is logical to conclude that the decision maker has already taken the steps necessary to gain authority for a decision. You also know from a previous discussion with the CIO that the Board needed to approve the recommendation of which company to choose and the Board met on July 25 ahead of the August 1 decision date. For that reason, we can logically eliminate Personal Ability as a factor leaving People Motivation and People Ability as the remaining two factors.

The third and final step of applying the Confluence Matrix is the most challenging and riskiest as we are close to forming the hypothesis. In our example, it is difficult to determine if a person is interfering with a decision which would be an indicator of People Motivation. For example, it is possible that the Chief of Staff for the hospital medical staff prefers a company different from the CIO. The CEO likely will listen to the CIO and give careful consideration to his or her recommendation. The CEO also cares about the support of the Chief of Staff.

To narrow to one factor, we consider what we know. Due to the risks associated with a bad decision as described previously, it is logical that the CEO desires cover, or said differently, the CEO desires to have consensus of the decision by the stakeholders. This allows others to share "ownership" of the decision with the CEO and reduces the Career Risk to the CEO. The delay could logically be related to a lack of consensus.

We also have reason to believe that there is not formal interference in the decision as we know the Board holds the authority for the decision and the CEO recommendation is likely key to their decision. It is not likely that the Board delayed a decision due to the looming deadlines. For that reason, I would gravitate to choosing the People Motivation factor as the likely factor affecting the lack of decision.

Therefore, our hypothesis related to the divide is: "A decision has not been made due to a potential lack of consensus among the stakeholders." This is logical based on our analysis to this point as consensus would create "cover" for the decision maker and therefore reduce the decision maker's Career Risk.

Now you must test the hypothesis by posing questions and gaining answers to these questions. Taking action on an unverified hypothesis is dangerous. You need to gain logical confidence that your theory is correct within the 90% threshold. In other words, gain enough information that you are 90% correct. That leads us to the next step in the sales strategy framework of Discovery Validation.

Discovery Validation. This step is just as it is named – you are working to discover information to validate your hypothesis. This involves two steps – posing appropriate questions, and then gaining data supported answers to those questions. Recall our discussion of the importance to avoid stacking assumptions. As part of this step, we need to test whether our assumptions that helped us form the hypothesis are correct and verifiable.

Posing and answering questions is often an art as much as a science. You may gain the correct answers but first you must choose the right questions to answer. For that reason, we recommend spending significant time developing the questions. This requires application of the emotional intelligence we discussed previously to remove your emotions and biases from the process. Proceeding "half cocked" or "half informed" can hurt your chances for success.

Related to our example hypothesis that Career Risk is a factor the issue causing the divide, we need to be open to the possibility that we had incomplete information. Related to this, the following are logical questions we might pose:

- Has any other event at the hospital diverted attention from the decision?
- Did the Board meet and take action as scheduled?
- Are the deadlines previously communicated still in place?

At this stage, I recommend reaching out to those that are the "dangerous people," or those that can say "no" but not "yes." These individuals are not likely to be your friends, but they have information that you need and likely can help your Discovery Validation process.

For our example of the EMR training company, you might reach out to the CIO, or one of their team members responsible for the implementation, and lead with probing questions. Proceed carefully and without accusations or threats. You may start with, "I know you have not made a decision but I am becoming increasingly concerned about the scheduled training timeline and delivering to your organization exceptional service. Do you know when a decision might be made?" Keep in mind that the the CIO probably has the same concerns you have.

Let's assume that the CIO shares with you that the CEO is getting push back from the Chief of Staff on the timeline for the implementation. The Chief of Staff would prefer for the implementation to occur in January rather than October and that is creating a conflict. The reason for the pushback is the timeline and not a disagreement among which company to choose. You also learn that you are still in the hunt to close the deal. What you have learned is invaluable as you have validated that the factor affecting the decision is in fact People Motivation. We know this as the information eliminates the other possibilities in the Confluence Matrix. Importantly, you do not have a reason to panic related to your company being chosen.

The strategy at this point is to be a resource to help close the deal. We have completed the steps of Define the Divide, Intelligent Speculation, and Discovery Validation. Now, you can formulate a plan to close the deal and hold the decision maker accountable to do so. More importantly, you are less likely to go in with one of the "half emotions." Your competition may not be so fortunate.

Now, we move to the final step of Closing the Deal. You know the issues that are prohibiting or delaying a decision by using the Accountability Sales strategy. The goal now is to Bridge the Divide by assisting the decision maker with closing the deal. Your job is not to fix the decision maker, force a decision, or dictate terms. Rather, think of yourself as a trusted advisor – you want the same thing the decision maker wants and that is to choose a solution that will solve the pain the decision maker is feeling. Your emotions are under control. You understand and you have validated the Divide. Now, Bridge the Divide to close the deal.

Bridging the Divide. Your goal here is to connect the decision maker with the solution you are selling. This is not about selling your services but reaching the decision finish line. We have formulated and validated our hypothesis and know what we need to do to hold the decision maker accountable to close the deal.

From our example, the timeline for implementation was chosen by the hospital. You did not choose it. Yes, they have missed their own decision date and to your knowledge the implementation date remains fixed. This causes a problem for your possible implementation plan. Unfortunately, you only have two choices: withdraw or get over it. This choice continues to require emotional intelligence.

It is possible that you are facing the necessity to withdraw your proposal as you do not believe you can provide the level of service that is important to you, and your reputation. Make this decision carefully as you may be walking away from earned business. Before you walk away, consider the differences in motivation and consequences.

Motivation versus Consequences. I remember a number of years ago the hospital where I was serving as CEO needed to purchase a replacement CT scanner. It was a large purchase and we had been balancing cash availability and praying our current scanner would not fail before it was replaced. We did have a secondary scanner so we could continue to provide the service, but capacity would be an issue.

I recall that we delayed the decision an extra sixty days as other more pressing issues took priority over that time period and our internal decision date was extended. The CT scanner sales professional was not happy. We had negotiated a price over a period of months and agreed to terms, but we had not committed to purchase.

I received an unannounced visit from the sales professional notifying me that if the decision took more than another 21 days, it would be necessary to return to the original price, not the price we had negotiated. So, I panicked and signed the deal right there. Well, that's not exactly what happened.

Actually, my reaction was an internal chuckle. I knew the sales professional would not walk away from the deal and I knew that the price would not increase. The 21 days was actually very logical as that was the end of a calendar quarter. I assumed it was possible that the sales professional had a quarterly quota, or even a bonus, and he needed the deal closed in the current quarter. Did I care? Nope.

So, what did I do? I waited not only 21 days but 30 days to sign the purchase agreement. There was no way I was going to sign the deal in the 21 days. Why did I do this? Quite frankly, because I could. The sales professional was playing a game of consequences and I found this offensive and inconsistent with how I preferred to conduct business. After the 30 days, I did sign the deal and the price did not increase from what we had negotiated. Shocker!

The above is an example of a failed sales strategy to close the deal using consequences. The attempt by the sales professional was to manipulate action but the tactic failed to achieve the desired result of the sales professional. The tactic was actually a deadline attached to a threat.

One of the early readers of this book, prior to publication, suggested that my above action to intentionally miss the dictated deadline was mean spirited. I have considered this and it concerned me that I might have acted with malice. Upon reflection, I do not believe I acted inappropriately. The sales professional was playing a game with the threat of consequences and I responded by playing the game he had begun. If a party in a negotiation plays a game, it is logical the other party will also play the game. This is the reason why consequences place you in a difficult position and should be avoided.

There are three types of consequences I have seen employed in sales. I refer to them as the "Deadly Ds" which include:

- Deadlines
- Demands
- Dazzle

Deadlines are just that – real or arbitrary drop dead dates to take action to close a deal. Unfortunately, as in our example, they rarely work unless a motivating factor is attached. Demands tend to be direct threats of action and resulting consequences. For example, a sales professional may state that if the decision maker does not make a decision to purchase an ultrasound machine from his or her company, then the company cannot give the decision maker a good price on the EKG machine next year.

Dazzle is where the sales professional attempts to "wow" you with their enthusiasm and likeability. No, that does not work. If a decision maker purchased from a particular sales professional just because they liked them, that decision maker was not necessarily considering the best interests of their organization. As a hospital CEO, I preferred to remain in a position where I was not swayed by a relationship. That said, I do like to do business with people I like and tend to avoid purchasing from those I do not like. Likeability and kindness are genuine. Dazzle is going too far by acting manipulative with self interest in mind.

The problem with consequences is they are not genuine. For that reason, they backfire as in my example of delaying a decision beyond the 21-day deadline. As a sales professional, unless the pain the decision maker is feeling is so significant to warrant a fast decision, they will make a decision when they want to do so. There is no amount of the "Deadly Ds" used in manipulation that will change the outcome.

Conversely, motivation works. Motivation is different from consequences in that it is genuine. You can motivate action when it has a positive impact on the decision maker and solving the pain they are feeling. As an example, a sales professional may share a fact that if the customer does not sign the purchase agreement this month, then they cannot guarantee installation of equipment next quarter. If that is genuine, it can be motivating if the decision maker feels some sense of urgency for installation in the next quarter. Or, a

149

sales professional can give the customer something that is of value in return for a faster decision. Both are examples of motivation and appropriate.

At this point in the Accountability Sales strategy steps, we have defined the divide, used intelligent speculation to form a hypothesis, and reasonably validated the hypothesis through discovery validation. We are ready to take the next step to closing the deal by proposing a solution.

Propose a Solution. Now that we have an understanding of the reason why a decision has not been made and the appropriate use of motivation versus consequences, you can move to propose a solution. The pain the decision maker feels is not subsiding and you know this. Your job is to become their ally and develop a solution to close the deal.

Returning to our example of the EMR Training, you know the hospital wants a successful implementation. More than likely, the implementation date was not chosen by the hospital but dictated at least partially by the EMR company. You also are reasonably confident that the delay in a decision is the implementation date debate with the Chief of Staff.

You desire to motivate a decision but not dictate terms by using consequences. You know that it takes you a minimum of three weeks lead time to line up resources for the EMR training. You also suspect that your competitor needs at least 30 days to line up resources. It is appropriate to craft a solution to motivate in the interest to act.

In our example, I recommend that you meet with the CIO, or his or her designee, and explain that you want nothing more than an implementation that has raving satisfaction of the physicians and staff trained on the new EMR. That is what they want and is good for you in the long run. You continue to explain that to achieve that goal, you need three weeks lead time to schedule your consultants. So, you propose a rolling 21-day implementation schedule. In other words, when the hospital makes a decision to select your company, you will be onsite in no more than 21 days to begin the training.

The typical response from the CIO would be to understand and accept that you have been honest and you are being flexible with what you can deliver. He or she will likely appreciate that you have expressed a desire for what is best for the hospital. Your goal is to arm the CIO with a solution and hope that they will now become your champion to carry your message to the decision maker.

A motivating solution leads to success through genuine recognition of your abilities and focusing on the needs of the company. You are focused on what matters. We now move to the final step in the Accountability Sales process of closing the deal.

Close the Deal. We have reached the final step in the Accountability Sales process where we actually close the deal. You should feel good but there is still work to be done. A phrase we commonly use in our training to explain your role in this step is, "Accountability – WTF?"

Many sales professionals view the finish line as the moment the agreement is signed. But, that is not "closing the deal." The agreement is signed but the solution is not implemented at a satisfactory level for all parties involved. More than likely, you would still prefer to be paid which is unlikely at the time the agreement is signed. The hospital would really like you to perform as promised.

Early in my work with Gylen Castle, we were sought out by a company that was struggling. They desperately needed a new Value Proposition Message and guidance in sales. They also needed significant management advisement related to strategic growth. As Gylen Castle was a relatively new company, this was a promising long term opportunity.

The agreement was signed and I started working immediately to put in place some changes that were desperately needed. Unfortunately, the partial advance payment to Gylen Castle was not delivered as promised within three days. After 10 days of work, I learned that the person that signed the agreement did not have the authority to commit the company to the deal. And, there were major disagreements among the directors of the company. I stopped working for the company. I still have a signed agreement but as of this writing, I have not been paid. It has only been 22 months since the agreement was signed – I am sure they are still good for it.

The point of the example is signing the agreement is not the finish line. The finish line is when both parties have delivered completely on the agreement terms. Your happiness, and your ongoing sales effectiveness, will both increase when you accept this to be true.

You have held the decision maker accountable to close the deal and they have signed the agreement but you still have work to do. You must hold the decision maker accountable to complete the deal using Accountability-WTF: Who, Timing, and Follow Up. What did you think WTF meant?

- *Who* will be responsible for implementation on the client side?
- What is the *Timing* for implementation and both parties meeting their obligations?
- Who will *Follow Up* to validate satisfaction by the client related to your company's performance?

When Accountability-WTF is completed and verified, you have now reached the finish line. Returning to our example, your strategy worked offering the rolling 21-day period for implementation. This was well received by the hospital leadership and your offer was a catalyst to achieving a favorable decision. Your company was selected and you crossed the finish line when training consultation was provided and your final payment received. In fact, you are now positioned to earn additional business from other hospitals in the same system.

Accountability Sales works when you are methodical in using data and following our process for closing deals. Yes, you can hold the decision maker accountable to help you close the deal but this requires both art and science in *Selling to the Pain*. More importantly, you should apply your own personal style to the process and focus on what matters – closing the deal.

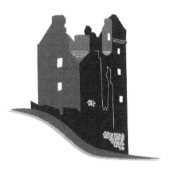

Chapter 12: What Do I Do Now?

This book was designed to challenge your way of thinking related to healthcare sales strategy. Again, I do not teach sales training as that must be personalized to your skill set. But, I do highly advocate a strong and efficient sales strategy rooted in The Decision Table and Accountability Sales. You must adapt a sales strategy for your company that is effective, efficient, and focused on what matters: closing more deals.

Selling to the Pain provides a solid strategy to adapt your culture to a consistent method of success. You now have the roadmap to *Selling to the Pain* to formulate your strategy and tools. The key, however, is the implementation. This requires that you invest in what you have learned.

As an author and reader, I encourage you to challenge what you have read and learned in this book. A number of years ago I read a book by Colin Powell related to leadership. It took me a year to read his book. The reason for the long time to complete the book is that periodically I would read a section of the book and I was not sure I agreed with his premise or conclusions. I would put down the book to consider if I agreed. When I made that decision, I would continue reading. I have great admiration for Powell but that does not mean I agree with everything he wrote.

I challenge you to do the same with *Selling to the Pain* as I did with Powell's book. Read and re-read this book, or sections of this book, and decide if you agree or disagree with my premises and conclusions. The right strategy for you is the strategy that leads improvement in your primary success metrics of Presentation Rate and Close Rate.

This final chapter includes two parts. First, I have provided a very brief summary of the principles of this book to provide a refresher now and in the future. In the coming months, I encourage you at a minimum to invest a few hours in reading this summary, re-reading portions of chapters of the book, and pondering your experiences over the prior weeks. Apply your understanding of decision making to evaluate real life instances of pain the clients are feeling and when Career Risk is at play. Most importantly, practice using Accountability Sales when working to close deals and consider how this is most effective for your style.

The second part of this chapter includes our recommendations for your next steps. These are commonly the standard next steps of our client engagements and should be tailored to your company culture and attributes. If you already have a recommended step covered, skip that step and move to the next. Application leads to success.

A Pithy Summary. Healthcare sales have become more difficult over the past two decades. Healthcare leaders are feeling increased pressure to balance performance in financial, satisfaction, and quality indicators. The culture of healthcare leadership has also changed. In the past, there were many Cowboy decision makers willing to take bold action in the decision process. Over time, this boldness has diminished due to a concern for Career Risk and a changing culture among c-suite leaders. Decision makers now rely more heavily on team members and committees to participate in the decision process to reduce perceived Career Risk and to be more inclusive of others. This has led to the rise of the most dangerous person to sell to – the person that can tell you "no" but not "yes."

Executives are also dealing with a lot of noise that causes distractions from making decisions. As a result, they experience difficulty sifting through the many opportunities presented to them and feel overwhelmed by the number of decisions that need to be made.

Understanding the decision process and the factors that influence decisions is a key to success. Using The Decision Table, an understanding of these factors helps you better navigate the sales process. The table includes four legs of financial performance, quality performance, satisfaction performance, and Career Risk the decision maker feels. These four areas not only impact the stability of the decision process but also influence which decisions will take priority. What decisions are made when can be predicted by the factors of The Decision Table.

It is also essential to understand your sales strategy and culture. Many company leaders do not realize the shifts in decision culture and the market influence and how these affect their sales strategy. They believe that if the strategy worked before, it will work again but that is not necessarily the case. The "try harder" strategy is often employed rather than a pivot in the sales strategy used. You cannot out hustle a mediocre sales strategy. To be effective and efficient in healthcare sales, you must learn *Selling to the Pain*.

The pain experienced in an organization is when performance is not reaching expected levels and a solution to improve performance is needed. In *Selling to the Pain*, you have identified the leg of The Decision Table that is creating the most concern for the organization. Once the pain is identified and defined, you can tailor a solution to solve the pain.

I recommend the use of a powerful Value Proposition Message to explain the value that your company creates for the client and the pain you solve. The Value Proposition Message is developed into three useful communication tools including the 60-Second Pitch, the One Pager, and the Discussion Presentation.

Once you have developed an understanding of the pain and the decision process, you are ready to close more deals. Accountability Sales is our unique way to navigate the decision process and hold the decision maker accountable to help you close the deal. Accountability Sales includes the following steps:

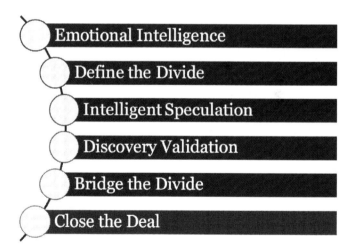

An element of Accountability Sales is use of the Confluence Matrix to understand the reasons why a decision is made or a decision is delayed. I recommend following our three step process to apply the Matrix to identify the reasons for decisions, or lack thereof. Once you know the reason, you can tailor a message for your solution to be acted upon.

	Motivation	Ability
Internal	Is the Decision Maker not motivated?	Does the Decision Maker have authority?
People	Does the Decision Maker require help or cover?	What person(s) are needed to help make a decision?
External	Is the Decision Maker dealing with competing demands?	What resources are needed?

What matters in your sales strategy is to close more deals. Application of *Selling to the Pain* will lead to improved performance in your Presentation Rate and Close Rate. Efficiency in your process is the key to success.

What do you do now? The best strategies are worthless without application and execution. *Selling to the Pain* is no different. The challenge you now face is to build a strategy for execution that will lead to success. Remember what matters – closing more deals. I recommend the below actions as your plan for implementation to effectively pivot your sales strategy when *Selling to the Pain*.

1. Complete an honest assessment to define your current sales strategy.

2. Assess the culture of your organization and evaluate if your culture is consistent with your sales strategy.

3. Adopt the critical success metrics of Presentation Rate and Close Rate and consistently measure your success rates.

4. Complete a margin analysis of your products and services. Are you focusing on those products and services that will drive your future success?

5. Define your services and products by what value they create for clients.

6. Identify the pain your solutions solve. You likely have multiple solutions to multiple pain points.

7. Define your prospective clients – who are your ideal clients, and not ideal clients, from the perspective of your margins and the efficiency of the various sales cycles?

8. Conduct a deep dive competitor analysis to understand where you are positioned in the market relative to competitors.

9. Invest in training for your team members that have sales responsibilities or provide support to sales.

This training should include *Selling to the Pain* and our core elements of Accountability Sales and The Decision Table.

10. Develop an effective Value Proposition Message and the related tools of the 60-second Pitch, One Pager, and Discussion Presentation following our guidelines.

11. Realign your marketing materials to be consistent with your Value Proposition Message and tools.

12. Finally, get out there and close more deals, more efficiently and more effectively.

I understand the above can be overwhelming. Pivoting your sales strategy and aligning your culture are large tasks even for the best leaders. The importance here is that you have a methodical approach to develop your strategy and then implement the strategy. Success is not achieved overnight.

The good news is this book has provided the materials needed to develop your effective adoption of the *Selling to the Pain* strategy. The better news is we are here to help. We have engagements available to advance your strategy in an advisory role, or we can lead your strategy design and execution. We can train your team, develop your Value Proposition Message, create the tools, and help you improve your culture related to sales. The best part is we customize all engagements to the client – we help you prioritize your needs and then provide what you need when you need it.

As I have said many times, you cannot out hustle a bad sales strategy. *Selling to the Pain* is not easy, but it is proven and effective.

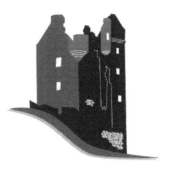

Section 4: Pearls of Wisdom

Section 4 of this book may feel a little disjointed from the rest of the book. That is intentional. This section is intended to address some sales myths and share some secondary thoughts on sales effectiveness. Yes, this information applies to the principles of this book but I really could not find the perfect place to share this information in the previous three sections. In the interest of efficiency, this is bonus time!

As explained previously, "Pearls of Wisdom" is a phrase borrowed from Chuck Beaman, CEO of Palmetto Health. I realized that my mentors had invaluable experience and knowledge that you just do not learn unless you sit at the feet of great leaders and you are smart enough to apply duct tape.

My personal Pearls of Wisdom have originated from various sources including people and experiences. As this book is about sales effectiveness, the chosen Pearls are related to our topic. Additionally, I will try to address some of the questions I am commonly asked during engagements. The topics will be disjointed so read these as short stories that are not connected.

In the words of Chuck Beaman, "...let me drop a Pearl on you."

Pearl #1: You Hired Who?

One of the most common questions I am asked is if it is better to hire a technical person or a professional sales person for a sales focused position. This assumes the position is selling a service or product that requires at least some technical understanding. Before I answer, there is not a clear, bold and unequivocal answer to this question that works for every company. However, as you may surmise after reading to this point, I do have an opinion.

What ultimately matters when hiring is not past sales performance but future anticipated performance of the candidates. I really do not give a lot of credence to past sales performance success unless the person was selling a substantially similar product to the same clients when they achieved that prior success. For example, a sales professional that moves from Smith & Nephew to Striker, competing orthopedic implant companies, would have a track record that would matter in the hiring decision process. But, if that same sales professional is changing from selling orthopedic implants to a software solution, we cannot assume past performance is an indicator of future performance. The difference is not only what they are selling but also the person to whom they are selling.

Further, a sales professional that is very successful in the past with a high touch relationship building sales approach will potentially struggle if they start selling a product in a low touch approach where relationships are not as important. The reason is the required sales skills and tactics are different.

The generation of the potential client is also a big issue here. Millennials and Gen Y-ers do not have as strong an interest in building a relationship in a business setting as do Baby Boomers. If you push too hard, the younger generations will disconnect. A sales professional can shift gears to adjust to client needs but you should not assume he or she will just do this without having to retrain his or her brain and develop a new strategy.

Personality is ultimately the key to sales success. If a sales professional is going to be successful, they have to be genuine. And, to be genuine, you have to have inherent personality traits that are necessary in sales. For example, a person that is not outgoing cannot fake being outgoing. Personality traits required to be successful in sales include friendly, confident, outgoing, kind, and genuinely interested in other people. You have to be a servant to sell effectively. This is necessary to truly care about helping to solve someone else's pain.

In the words of Ron White, "You cannot fix stupid." Unfortunately, an unintelligent person has difficulty grasping highly detailed topics and learning at a deep level. I learned this the hard way. I hired a former pharmaceutical sales professional to be a Physician Liaison at one of my hospitals. She had a proven track record in sales and had the personality traits that I thought were necessary. I thought I made a good hire. I was wrong.

The problem was this person had been really good at having a deep understanding of a few pharmaceuticals. As an analogy, she was 100 feet deep over about a one-foot span of knowledge. Now as a Physician Liaison for many different physician specialties using the various services of the hospital, she had a new challenge. We expected her to be 20 feet deep over a 100-foot span of knowledge regarding the complexities of hospital operations. This was very difficult for her to adapt and develop a wide understanding. She was not a dumb person and actually very intelligent. But, she could not handle what was expected of her and I missed the differences in the two roles.

Technical sales skills are also required in addition to the necessary personality traits. You need the skill set to effectively listen to others, navigate negotiations, and communicate. These are technical skills that can be learned. It is also helpful for the sales professional to be intelligent enough to understand how your service or product works so that he or she can match your sales pitch to the need that exists.

If a sales professional is selling a technology solution such as equipment or software, he or she needs to have a technical background or at least the ability to learn the technical knowledge. You cannot fake understanding the technology behind your solution. The reason is the client is likely to be reasonably knowledgeable of the problem and the solution and they will quickly identify if the sales professional does not have a working knowledge. That said, if a person has the ability to learn the technology they do not necessarily need to have a technological background or skill set. Applied knowledge is the key whether this is from education or experience.

Most important to your hire is the team members must have adequate training. These team members need an understanding of the company culture, the clients, the solutions, and the company sales strategy. On an individual basis, depending on the background of the sales professional and the type of company in which they are working, there is a need for technical training or sales training.

Don't skip the sales training regardless of the person or situation. Otherwise, it is so much harder to get a return on your investment in your sales professionals. The bottom line is this – hire those that have the skills you cannot teach and teach the skills that can be taught. You cannot teach someone to be outgoing, driven, aggressive, determined, driven, or kind. But, if they have these traits, you can teach them the art and science of sales and your solutions.

Hire wisely when choosing your sales professionals. It is one of the most important decisions a company makes in terms of impact on their future. Once hired, invest in them to assure your return on investment.

Pearl #2: Culture Eats Strategy for Lunch

You have probably heard this one before, but my take on this phrase if related to sales strategy. Many ignore company culture and how it affects sales strategy effectiveness. Companies spend an inordinate amount of time focusing on strategy without consideration for culture. Culture should be addressed first. Seek first to understand your culture and then you can leverage the culture to achieve your goals.

During a typical Executive Connections Engagement with Gylen Castle, I interview those who have a role in sales for our client companies. This includes some enlightening discussions that are not necessarily a surprise to me but some of the information surprises the leadership. This is commonly due to the fact that leaders run at such a rapid pace they do not slow down long enough to assess their culture. Worse than that, they assume they understand their culture, and, more concerning, their understanding is inaccurate.

When interviewing a team for one client, I realized the company had a potential issue. The team was very congruent in their vision, drive, and personality. Well, the team was congruent except for the newest sales team member. He had a different view of sales and exuded an almost irrational confidence in his ability to sell.

I was not concerned about his overconfidence. My concern was he was not in sync with the culture of the organization related to other team members. This can cause some real problems. I do not know how long the new team member lasted with the company but I hope he has succeeded. The concern I had was the potential damage to the effective culture that was already in place and proving successful. One bad team member can do a lot of damage to progress and growth.

To protect and grow your company, focus on first understanding your culture and then leveraging those strengths to grow your business. Strategy is important but culture trumps strategy every time. Your sales strategy may be outstanding but will only be effective if aligned with your culture.

Our engagements improve your culture and strategy and it is important to assess and address both. The leaders and the teams are very interested in our findings and recommendations related to culture. We recommend that you carefully study your culture, implement the necessary tweaks, and then develop *Selling to the Pain* around your culture.

Pearl #3: Don't Boil the Ocean

During my time working on my Doctorate degree, I had to write a Dissertation related to a statistical research study I designed and performed. I was terrified by the challenge. Part of my fear was due to my lack of knowledge related to statistics. We had three statistics courses in our curriculum. Using a prior analogy in Pearl #2, my knowledge was an inch deep and a mile wide regarding all of the different statistical tests and their applications to study data.

The other part of my fear was related to designing a Dissertation that I could wrap my head and hands around. A Dissertation is a research study which is attached to management theory. Some also refer to Dissertations as Theses.

Prior to selecting my topic, I was very interested in whether or not informed patients could help a hospital improve performance. Unfortunately, that is a very broad topic that needed to be narrowed.

A Dissertation is commonly 80-200 pages and includes 30,000 to 60,000 words. I was not writing a 200-page Dissertation. I also was not creating a research study that had dozens of different statistical tests. For this paper, I needed to go 100 feet deep in a one-foot-wide portion of statistical knowledge.

I decided to take the advice of one of my professors, "don't boil the ocean." What he meant was you have to narrow your research study to something you can reasonably boil such as a large pot of water. I needed to reduce my Dissertation topic to something I could get in a "pot" and had manageable statistical testing.

I always had an interest in Emergency Department operations and I had a deep appreciation for how this department impacted the entire hospital. A bad Emergency Department could affect every department in the hospital. I also realized that by focusing on Emergency Department efficiency the hospital could drive efficiency improvement across the organization due to the inter-dependencies of the various departments.

As a hospital CEO, my teams implemented a lot of Emergency Department improvement strategies including constructing facilities, improving patient flow, retooling staffing, and even adding integrated services. We did achieve a lot of efficiency improvement but we eventually reached a plateau and could not continue to improve. Our emphasis had been exclusively internal strategies and we eventually had to turn to external strategies to continue our improvement trend.

The most common problem of Emergency Department inefficiency was related to when patient volumes were not as expected. This could include times when the department was overcrowded with more patients than expected. Inefficiency was also present when we did not have enough patients for the resources allocated. As a result, there was a narrow range in volumes at any given time of the day when our patient volume matched our resources available. When volumes did not match resources, our operations were inefficient.

As I left the Emergency Department one day during a period of overcrowding, I laughed to myself that our problems would be resolved if I could get the patients to show up to the Emergency Department at the right times. I stopped walking. What if we could engage patients in decision making that would help the hospital? In other words, how could we encourage more patients to arrive to the Emergency Department when volumes were low and fewer patients to arrive to the Emergency Department when volumes were high? This strategy to improve efficiency would be external and relate to patient engagement thus improving performance.

My research took me to theory and I studied carefully Rational Choice Theory. This theory is rooted in science that informed consumers will make rational choices of when to purchase a service or good compared to alternatives. The consumer will act based on available information and act in self interest, or in other words, they will choose to purchase the product or service that is perceived to be best for them. A sub theory of Rational Choice Theory is Bounded Rationality whereby a consumer will not search out information indefinitely but will eventually believe they have enough information to make a decision. The bounded element is the consumer stops looking for additional information.

Returning to our Emergency Department issue, the patient did not know when the Emergency Department had low volumes or high volumes. They did not know this information because we did not tell them. As a result, the patient did not have the information to act rationally and that needed to change.

I explored multiple strategies to share wait times in the Emergency Department with patients including posting current wait times on billboards, the hospital website, text messaging, and mobile apps. I also explored reservation systems where the patient could make an appointment to arrive at the hospital at a time provided by the hospital. I was intrigued by the alternatives.

This same concept of "don't boil the ocean" applies in sales strategy. Many companies make the mistake of offering too many services or products. You cannot be all to all. What many of you are thinking now is that is not a problem for your company. But, unless you are a major exception, you also have too many services or products. You must carefully determine your offerings and not "boil the ocean."

The bottom line is this – potential clients will hire you, or purchase from you, if they believe you are the best. To be the best, you must be viewed as an expert. Unfortunately, potential clients will not view you as an expert of a lot of different things. For that reason, I recommend narrowing your focus of services or products and work on achieving expert status. By so doing, you will find greater efficiency and long term success.

You may recall from earlier in this book that Gylen Castle had grown and extended well beyond the healthcare client base where we held expertise. By returning to a narrower niche focus on companies selling to healthcare organizations, we were able to grow our revenue. This was due to the real and perceived expertise of our leadership.

Don't boil the ocean. Narrow your services and products to achieve expertise and a reputation as the best in your space.

For those who are interested in my Dissertation research and findings, I provided the abstract of the Dissertation below and a link to the full published research study in the References section of this book.

Abstract of Dissertation:

Emergency Department Communication Strategies and
Patient Throughput Efficiency
McDougal, O'Connor, Booth, Hearld, and Landry (2015)

This study investigates hospital strategies used to inform patients of anticipated wait times in the Emergency Department (ED) and the association of such strategies with patient throughput efficiency. When hospitals are inefficient in ED patient throughput, conditions of overcrowding often occur. Overcrowding of the ED is a problem for many hospitals. When such conditions exist, there is evidence in the literature that it leads to lower patient satisfaction, care quality, and financial position of the hospital. Therefore, improving patient throughput efficiency is a priority for hospitals.

To improve patient throughput efficiency, hospitals use a variety of strategies. This study focuses on two wait time communication strategies of posting ED wait times on the hospital website and the use of ED reservation systems. Through application of Rational Choice Theory, it is expected that patients who are informed of anticipated wait times will make rational decisions related to visiting a potentially overcrowded ED. Thus, engaged patients make decisions that can contribute to improved ED efficiency.

The question of this research study is "Do ED wait time communication strategies improve patient throughput efficiency?" This study sample includes acute care hospitals in Florida and the ED throughput efficiency metrics from the Center for Medicare and Medicaid Services (CMS) Hospital Compare data sets to contrast the performance of hospitals that use the study strategies.

The results of the study indicate that posting ED wait times on the hospital website has a statistically significant association with ED efficiency. However, the use of reservation systems does not have a statistically significant association with ED efficiency. Further, the control variables of hospital licensed bed size, metropolitan location, percent of population without health insurance, and percent of population Medicaid eligible have a statistically significant association with ED efficiency.

Consistent with expected behavior related to Rational Choice Theory, this study supports that informed patients will make logical decisions related to if and when to visit an ED for care and therefore contribute to improved throughput efficiency. (McDougal, O'Connor, Booth, Hearld, and Landry, 2015)

Pearl #4: You Ain't Jesus

In Chapter 1, I shared one of my favorite stories from my days as a hospital CEO. This story involved Karen, our Chief Nursing Officer, and the hospital weekend nursing supervisor handling an emergency department patient that had left without treatment. So you do not have to return to Chapter 1, this is a summary of the story:

> *On a Monday morning, our Chief Nursing Officer, Karen, came into my office and was not in her normal happy mood as she needed to inform me of an incident over the weekend. We had a large psych unit and a patient had arrived in the ER with some psychiatric issues and needed admitting. But, the staff had turned their backs for just a moment and the patient had slipped out the back door and eloped into the community.*

The weekend Nursing Supervisor was one of the best I had ever worked with but that night she made a mistake and left the hospital to help the police find the patient. Karen was fuming and I asked her what she had said to the supervisor. Karen said, "I told her, 'you ain't Jesus!'" I could not stop laughing. Karen explained that the statement was an order that the supervisor's job is to look out for the many patients in the hospital, not the one patient that left. Of course, this was a reference to the Bible, Matthew 18:12-14.

In Pearl #3, we talked about "don't boil the ocean" recognizing the importance of narrowing your focus in products and services to be an expert in the field for a narrow niche. In this pearl, we focus on "you ain't Jesus", but with a twist.

Converse to Karen's advice, you should take the advice of Jesus. Worry about the one, not the many. As I shared with you, Gylen Castle was formed for multiple purposes including general consulting. I actually had a pretty strong book of business in consulting and did not mind the work. I eventually decided I didn't like the work that much when I did a deep dive and realized just how low our margins were for general consulting. The reason was simple – competition.

Just about anyone with special information or experience can be a consultant. In fact, you are a consultant if someone is willing to pay you for work you do in which they find value based on your ability or expertise. With so many consultants, it was hard to differentiate Gylen Castle from the crowd as a general management and leadership consulting firm. In our early years, Gylen Castle took on projects and work inside and outside of healthcare and I rarely turned down work. But, I realized we eventually had strayed from our purpose. More concerning, we had strayed from our expertise. Just because we were experts in healthcare did not mean that would translate to accounting, education, manufacturing, law, or banking. In fact, our expertise in healthcare limited our reputation in other fields.

I considered broadening our resources and team to continue to focus on other industries outside of healthcare. Marketing materials and our website were expanded. Then one day I reached a point that the website was a mess. We were trying to be everything to everyone and it was not working. Rather than panicking, I returned the company to its core emphasis of healthcare. We focused on a narrow niche of clients that really found value in our expertise. The result was that our revenues grew rather than declined. The moral of the story is "Be Jesus." Focus on a narrow client base of the one rather than the many.

Pearl #5: Players in the Decision Process

As shared in Chapter 6, the players in the decision process of hospitals have a significant amount of influence. The influence is impacted by a variety of factors related to the hospital characteristics and the delegation of authority. When navigating the decision process, it is a good suggestion to have some understanding of the players and common tendencies. You may recall that the three defining factors of individual power regardless of role are authority, influence, and how they roll.

This is the section of the book that will get me in trouble. Stereotyping will do that. Please grant me some grace in this section as it is intended to offer a glimpse into leadership functions within hospitals and not a statement of quality, ability, or skill of these individuals based on their title. My opinions of generalities and tendencies are only intended to be my opinions. And, it is certainly not a reflection of my opinions of individuals with whom I have or will work.

Keep in mind that if you have seen one hospital leader, you have seen one hospital leader. But, they do have some common tendencies that when understood will help you navigate the decision process.

These leadership positions are evaluated on the three characteristics of authority, influence, and "how they roll" related to their inclusiveness of others in their activities and decision involvement.

COO, Vice Presidents, and Assistant Administrators. These positions are discussed together as the tendencies are the same. There is no other position in the c-suite that varies so greatly between hospitals in terms of consistency of authority, experience, autonomy, and decision making. In fact, the tendencies are difficult to address.

Generally, these leaders have the trust and listening ear of the CEO but they do not have decision authority. They can be your ally or a hindrance to get your message to the CEO for a decision. The good news is if you can sell these individuals on taking your idea to the CEO, you likely do have an ally.

COOs and Assistant CEOs in small to midsize for-profit hospital tend to be on a career track and are extremely sensitive to

Career Risk. If you can position your sales approach with these individuals in a way so that their perception of Career Risk is low and the opportunity for positive recognition is high, you are more likely for these individuals to recommend your solution to the decision maker.

Age is a factor with these positions as well. Older individuals with these titles tend to be extremely seasoned operators who make good well-calculated decisions. Younger leaders tend to have a different generational approach. For these reasons, as a general rule, use a high touch sales approach with the older leaders and a low touch approach with the younger leaders. High touch is a relationship building approach where you and the leader communicate regularly and at a deeper level. Conversely, a low touch approach is a more distant communication and the relationship is not as important.

Chief Financial Officer. The Chief Financial Officer of the organization is generally a powerful individual. Experience level and skill set varies greatly depending on the ownership type. For-profit systems with large corporate offices tend to have more structured and centralized functions and expectations. For this reason, the CFO functions in a well defined calendar and format. While they are very intelligent individuals, they tend to be stronger on income statement functions than balance sheet functions. And, they have limited current working knowledge of treasury and financing functions. None of this is suggesting lack of intelligence or experience but a statement that their functions are more limited due to the environment. The above is also true for large non-profit systems where the balance sheet and treasury work are centralized in the system office.

Regarding authority, the CFO generally has relatively limited authority. They definitely have the ear of the CEO but the CEO normally retains the authority for decision making. Regarding supply chain and revenue cycle functions, the CEO will normally default to the CFO's views and opinions but the authority remains with the CEO.

In my opinion, the CFO has the hardest job in the c-suite. They must not only accept responsibility and accountability for a very difficult industry environment but they must also understand how financial decisions impact quality and satisfaction metric outcomes. The best of the best do this extremely well. CEOs and the COO/VP/Assistant Administrator group seem to have a more balanced view of all metric performances including financial but the CFO just has to make more effort to avoid a myopic view point.

Regarding support from their team, the CFO is generally very reliant on the persons that are leading the Revenue Cycle and Supply Chain functions. As the CFO has the ear of the CEO, these leaders have the ear of the CFO. For that reason, they commonly work closely together on decisions related to these important functions.

Chief Nursing Officer. The clinical functions of the hospital are normally split with nursing functions reporting to the CNO while ancillary departments generally report to the COO or a Vice President. This can create some silo effects unless the leaders have a strong desire to work together. For this reason, the COO or CEO is sometimes required to pull the functions together for consensus.

CNOs generally have worked their way through the ranks and eventually promoted up the ladder to the CNO role. For this reason, they tend to have strong clinical knowledge and have one or two areas of nursing where they are consciously, or subconsciously, more experienced and partial. For example, if a CNO has a strong background in ICU, they will be more oriented towards this department.

As a very significant stereotype from my experience, the CNO's primary duty is to assemble and lead a team of very good nursing department managers. CNOs spend most of their time in support of these individuals and are very policy and procedure oriented as that is the glue that holds the organization together. The best of the best are improvement oriented and always searching for innovative ideas. But, adoption of these innovations is normally slow as they tend to want to implement solutions that are proven.

In terms of authority, the CNO has enormous authority related to day-to-day operations but limited authority for implementing significant change. Regarding contracting, the CNO rarely has authority to enter into contracts.

Chief Quality Officer. The leader of the quality operations of the hospital are generally deferred and entrusted to the Quality Director or the Chief Quality Officer (CQO). While the titles can vary, I will refer to all quality leaders as the CQO. These individuals tend to perform their duties on an island where they have been granted a certain amount of autonomy of prioritized duties but they do not carry contracting authority.

The largest challenge with CQOs is they generally have a different perspective than the rest of the c-suite. CQOs are focused on patient care and are very interested in the patient care indicators and patient satisfaction outcomes. I have noticed a tendency that the average CQO is very strong on reporting but not as strong on implementing change unless the c-suite is pushing for change. For this reason, the culture of the c-suite usually dictates the aggressiveness of the CQO. If the CEO is very focused on improving quality, the CQO tends to carry more authority and act more aggressively. Regarding dotted line supervisory authority to department managers by the CQO, the authority is earned by performance and reputation and what is granted from the CEO.

The CQO tends to be very team and committee oriented. They seek teamwork as they need the support to monitor performance and implement change, and welcome opinions and input. The reality is that most hospitals still struggle with tracking quality performance metrics as operational software in hospitals are not strong in this area.

The relationship between CNO and CQO is very important to an organization. A strong relationship is expected to result in better quality and satisfaction performance. There are times that the COO or CEO have to arbitrate disagreements between CQO and CNO but these are not typical.

Chief Information Officer. This individual typically has the title of Chief Information Officer (CIO), Director of Information Systems, or sometimes Chief Technology Officer. Regardless, they function the same. However, a director level position obviously will have less influence than a c-suite level position. Regarding authority, the CIO typically does not have contract authority.

These individuals generally have a significant amount of power in an organization. As technology innovation has risen, the autonomy and size of the Information Technology (IT) team has not grown proportionally. For that reason, resources are typically limited and that creates power for the CIO as they can greatly influence what projects will be completed and when. This leads to a generally slow implementation timeline for IT projects that do not have the highest priority.

Part of the reason for the implementation challenges is the type of personnel resources available to the CIO. I personally experienced in multiple organizations that the balance between software and hardware individual expertise was a challenge. The CIO builds and maintains a team but different initiatives require a different software/hardware mix of expertise. If you are implementing a software solution but your IT department is heavy on hardware personnel, resources can be an issue.

For the reasons above, while the CIO has limited contracting authority, they have great power related to implementation. Most importantly, the COO, CFO, and CEO listen to them.

Supply Chain Directors. These individuals are powerful in an organization and generally report to the CFO. They have challenges on a daily basis to manage inventory and to make sure the organization has the resources it needs when it needs them. But, they also have pressure to keep costs to a minimum. They are influenced by the Group Purchasing Organization (GPO) that the hospital uses. Previously, I addressed the impact of GPOs on the decision process.

In terms of authority, the Supply Chain Director typically has authority granted to them associated with limitation of purchases. These limitations are often restricted to work within a budgeted amount and purchase from GPO vendors and to maintain inventory levels. If an organization is "off contract," meaning they are not part of the GPO approved vendors, the Supply Chain Director commonly has his or her hands tied.

That said, the Supply Chain Director has significant influence with the CFO and they work together closely. The Supply Chain Director is one of the most powerful persons that can tell you "no," but not yes. The other person with this type of influence is the Revenue Cycle Director.

Revenue Cycle Director. These individuals typically carry the title of Revenue Cycle Director (RCD) or Business Office Director. One significant distinguishing factor is the RCD typically has more influence over the Medical Records Department than a Business Office Director, which includes the insurance reimbursement coding functions. This is a significant differentiator. However, all functions ultimately are managed by the CFO.

The RCD commonly has significant influence but very limited authority. As they control the collection of money, the c-suite listens to them. Typically, this is a thankless job and I would often refer to them as the center on the football offensive line. If they are doing their job, they do not get a lot of attention. But, if there are issues, they are noticed. The expectation is high performance all the time and that creates a significant amount of pressure and can be a distraction. Talented RCDs are invaluable to the organization. As with others that report to the CFO, the RCD tends to have a lot of oversight and work more in a silo without a lot of team work functions outside of their department.

RCDs also tend to have climbed the ladder similar to CNOs. For that reason, their background often dictates their specific area of expertise and emphasis on performance.

Contact Information

Gylen Castle is here to meet your needs. To learn more about our training and implementation strategies, contact us today to explore a customized approach to improving your sales strategy to close more deals. Chapter 12 included a list of recommended steps to shape your strategy to implement *Selling to the Pain*. We are anxious to explore how we can help. Our contact information is below for your reference and we welcome an opportunity to discuss how you can increase your close rates in the challenging environment of healthcare sales.

Tom R. McDougal, Jr. D.Sc., MSHA, MBA, FACHE
CEO and Founder
Gylen Castle, LLC
22 Inverness Center Parkway, Suite 160
Birmingham, Alabama 35242
info@gylencastle.com
205-215-3060

References

Cain, B. *Toilets, Bricks, Fish Hooks and Pride: The Peak Performance Toolbox Exposed.* (2013) 2nd Edition. Quality Books.

McDougal, T., O'Connor, S., Booth, S., Hearld, K., and Landry, A. (2015) *Emergency Wait Time Communication Strategies and Patient Throughput Efficiency.* ProMed.
http://gradworks.umi.com/37/19/3719220.html

Patterson, K., Grenny, J., McMillan, R., Switzler, A., & Maxfield, D. (2013). *Crucial Accountability: Tools for Resolving Violated Expectations, Broken Commitments, and Bad Behavior,* (Paperback). McGraw-Hill Professional.

Selling to the Pain

Closing More Deals in Healthcare Sales

Dr. Tom R. McDougal, Jr.
CEO and Founder
Gylen Castle, LLC

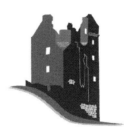

43991137R00118

Made in the USA
San Bernardino, CA
03 January 2017